# Pediatric Orthopedics

*Editor*

MARK E. SOLOMON

# CLINICS IN PODIATRIC MEDICINE AND SURGERY

www.podiatric.theclinics.com

*Consulting Editor*
THOMAS J. CHANG

January 2022 • Volume 39 • Number 1

**ELSEVIER**

1600 John F. Kennedy Boulevard • Suite 1800 • Philadelphia, Pennsylvania, 19103-2899

http://www.theclinics.com

**CLINICS IN PODIATRIC MEDICINE AND SURGERY Volume 39, Number 1**
**January 2022 ISSN 0891-8422, ISBN-13: 978-0-323-85019-3**

Editor: Lauren Boyle
Developmental Editor: Diana Grace Ang

*Clinics in Podiatric Medicine and Surgery* (ISSN 0891-8422) is published quarterly by Elsevier Inc., 360 Park Avenue South, New York, NY 10010-1710. Months of issue are January, April, July, and October. Business and Editorial Offices: 1600 John F. Kennedy Blvd., Ste. 1800, Philadelphia, PA 19103-2899. Customer Service Office: 3251 Riverport Lane, Maryland Heights, MO 63043. Periodicals postage paid at New York, NY and additional mailing offices. Subscription prices are $319.00 per year for US individuals, $773.00 per year for US institutions, $100.00 per year for US students and residents, $393.00 per year for Canadian individuals, $796.00 for Canadian institutions, $476.00 for international individuals, $796.00 per year for international institutions, $100.00 per year for Canadian students/residents, and $220.00 per year for foreign students/residents. To receive student/resident rate, orders must be accompanied by name of affiliated institution, date of term, and the *signature* of program/residency coordinator on institution letterhead. Orders will be billed at individual rate until proof of status is received. Foreign air speed delivery is included in all *Clinics* subscription prices. All prices are subject to change without notice. POSTMASTER: Send address changes to *Clinics in Podiatric Medicine and Surgery*, Elsevier Health Sciences Division, Subscription Customer Service, 3251 Riverport Lane, Maryland Heights, MO 63043. **Customer Service: 1-800-654-2452 (US). From outside of the US, call 314-447-8871. Fax: 314-447-8029. E-mail: JournalsCustomerService-usa@elsevier.com (for print support); JournalsOnlineSupport-usa@elsevier.com (for online support).**

*Reprints.* For copies of 100 or more of articles in this publication, please contact the Commercial Reprints Department, Elsevier Inc., 360 Park Avenue South, New York, NY 10010-1710. Tel.: 212-633-3874; Fax: 212-633-3820; E-mail: reprints@elsevier.com.

*Clinics in Podiatric Medicine and Surgery* is covered in *MEDLINE/PubMed (Index Medicus)* and *EMBASE/Excerpta Medica*.

# Contributors

## CONSULTING EDITOR

**THOMAS J. CHANG, DPM**
Clinical Professor and Past Chairman, Department of Podiatric Surgery, California College of Podiatric Medicine, Faculty, The Podiatry Institute, Redwood Orthopedic Surgery Associates, Santa Rosa, California

## EDITOR

**MARK E. SOLOMON, DPM**
Director, The Pediatric Orthopedic Fellowship, Cedar Knolls, New Jersey

## AUTHORS

**AAMIR AHMED, DPM, AACFAS**
Ankle and Foot Doctors of New Jersey, Millburn, New Jersey

**TAMIR BLOOM, MD**
The Pediatric Orthopedic Center, Cedar Knolls, New Jersey

**MARYELLEN P. BRUCATO, DPM, FACFAS**
Brucato Foot and Ankle Surgery, Owner, Brucato Foot and Ankle Surgery, LLC, Clifton, New Jersey

**MATTHEW B. DOBBS, MD**
Dobbs Clubfoot Center, Paley Orthopaedic and Spine Institute, West Palm Beach, Florida

**LUCIAN M. FERARU, DPM**
Fellow, The Pediatric Orthopedic Fellowship, Cedar Knolls, New Jersey

**GAN GOLSHTEYN, MS, DPM**
Foot and Ankle Fellow, The Pediatric Orthopedic Center, Cedar Knolls, New Jersey

**HAYLEY E. IOSUE, DPM, AACFAS**
Surgical Fellow, University Hospitals Richmond Medical Center, Richmond Heights, Ohio

**ANNA KATSMAN, MD**
The Pediatric Orthopedic Center, Cedar Knolls, New Jersey

**DAVID Y. LIN, MD, FAAOS**
Pediatric Orthopedic Surgeon/Partner/Owner, The Pediatric Orthopedic Center, Cedar Knolls, New Jersey

**MARK J. MENDESZOON, DPM, FACFAS, FACFOAM**
Fellowship Director, Podiatric Surgery, University Hospitals Regional Hospitals Advanced Foot and Ankle Surgery Fellowship, Richmond Heights, Ohio

**MARK A. RIEGER, MD**
The Pediatric Orthopedic Center, Cedar Knolls, New Jersey

**SANJEEV SABHARWAL, MD, MPH**
Professor of Clinical Orthopaedics, Director, UCSF Pediatric Orthopaedic Fellowship, University of California, San Francisco, San Francisco, California; Director, Limb Lengthening and Reconstruction Center, UCSF Benioff Children's Hospital, Oakland, California

**HARRY P. SCHNEIDER, DPM**
Program Director, Department of Surgery, Cambridge Health Alliance, Assistant Professor of Surgery, Harvard Medical School, Cambridge, Massachusetts

**ALEXIS SCHUPP, DPM**
Fellow, University of Maryland Limb Preservation and Deformity Correction Fellowship, Baltimore, Maryland

**MARK E. SOLOMON, DPM**
Director, The Pediatric Orthopedic Fellowship, Cedar Knolls, New Jersey

**JOSHUA STRASSBERG, MD, FAAOS**
The Pediatric Orthopedic Center, Cedar Knolls, New Jersey

**JACOB WYNES, DPM, MS**
Assistant Professor, Department of Orthopaedics, University of Maryland School of Medicine, Program Director, University of Maryland Limb Preservation and Deformity Correction Fellowship, Baltimore, Maryland

**WILLIAM R. YORNS Jr, DO**
Department of Neurology, Assistant Professor of Pediatrics, UCONN School of Medicine, Connecticut Children's Medical Center, Farmington, Connecticut

# Contents

 Video content accompanies this article at http://www.podiatric.
theclinics.com/.

> Clubfoot or talipes equinovarus deformity is one of the most common
> anomalies affecting the lower extremities. This review provides an update
> on the outcomes of various treatment options used to correct clubfoot.
> The ultimate goal in the treatment of clubfoot is to obtain a fully functional
> and pain-free foot and maintain a long-term correction. The Ponseti
> method is now considered the gold standard of treatment for primary club-
> foot. Relapse is common after primary treatment with the Ponseti method,
> and other interventions are discussed that are used to provide for long-
> term successful outcomes.

> The neurologic causes of foot and leg dysfunction are reviewed. Disorders
> causing foot and ankle pain, weakness, or other sensorimotor distur-
> bances often cause difficulty with ambulation and prompt patients to
> seek medical evaluation. Physical signs and symptoms along with tar-
> geted diagnostic testing are needed to come to the correct diagnosis
> and treatment plan. An overview of peripheral nerve, muscle, and central
> nervous system disorders affecting the foot and leg are discussed.

> Children with cerebral palsy (CP) are at a high risk of developing foot and
> ankle deformities that can impact function, brace/shoe fit, and seating. The
> 3 commonly observed foot and ankle segmental malalignment patterns
> include equinus, planovalgus, and equinovarus. Assessment of foot defor-
> mities is multifaceted, requiring the collection and integration of data from
> a combination of sources that include the clinical history, standardized
> physical examination, observational and quantitative gait analysis,
> GMFCS classification, and radiographic findings. Surgical procedures
> are determined by identifying all segmental malalignments and assessing
> the contribution of dynamic or flexible soft-tissue imbalance, fixed soft-
> tissue imbalance, and skeletal deformities.

Musculoskeletal injuries of the lower limb are frequent in pediatric patients and represent the most common cause of emergency department admissions. Acute sports-related injuries commonly involve the lower extremity, as the knee and ankle are the most frequently injured parts. Physeal fractures are common injuries in children and adolescents participating in contact sports, which may lead to growth disturbances and cause limb length discrepancy. It is imperative for pediatric trauma centers to implement evidence-based multispecialty protocols for the perimanagement of the injured child, especially through the postdischarge and rehabilitation phases, in order for the child to resume active daily living.

This article explores different pediatric forefoot deformities including syndactyly, polydactyly, macrodactyly, curly toe, and congenital hallux varus. The epidemiology and genetic background are reviewed for each condition. Preferred treatment options and recommended surgical techniques are discussed with review of the current literature.

Recreational sports are more popular, with many athletes involved year-round in multiple sports and on multiple teams. Most athletes do not take proper rest, making them more susceptible to stress-related injuries. There are numerous sports-related injuries in the foot and ankle. These issues can be non-traumatic, due to chronic repetitive stresses, or traumatic. Most of these injuries are managed conservatively, and athletes do well and return to play, while some do better with operative management. This article discusses a few of the sports injuries that are common in the leg, foot, and ankle and the recovery process.

OCDs of the ankle are the third most common lesion in the body and a physician should include this in the differential while evaluating the pediatric population with the history of injury and/or pain in the ankle. Pain, stiffness, and swelling are the most common presenting complaints about the pediatric and adolescent patients with an OCD. Conservative treatment options should be attempted before attempting surgical intervention. Multiple surgical procedures exist to manage the lesion based on location, size, and other factors.

Jacob Wynes and Alexis Schupp

Limb length inequality or discrepancy (LLD) occurs when there is a difference in length between 2 limbs or when deviation exists from a normally
expected length for a given age. The magnitude of the discrepancy is
defined as the difference between the 2 extremities. Aside from congenital
etiologies, LLD can also arise from infection, paralysis, tumors/neoplasm,
and surgery. Approximately 70% to 90% of the world's population has
some elements of LLD with compensation allowing for tolerance and
potentially masking the extent to which one limb could be significantly
shorter either functionally or structurally. Components of functional LLD
could include congenital shortening of soft tissues, joint contractures, axial
skeleton malalignment, and abnormal pedal biomechanics (ie, posterior
tibial tendonitis or equinovarus). In accordance with literature reports,
most individuals can tolerate upwards of a 2 cm discrepancy. Although
a constellation of symptoms such as joint pain, arthritis, alterations in oxygen consumption/heart rate, and low back pathology can occur later on
in adulthood, the focus in this review will be with early diagnosis and management in the pediatric population.

Gan Golshteyn and Harry P. Schneider

Tarsal coalitions are recognized as a congenital anomaly whereby the two
or more bones of the hindfoot and midfoot are fused resulting in limitation
of foot motion and pain. Tarsal coalitions were found to be the cause of
painful flatfeet in adolescents and young adults. Developing a clinical understanding of tarsal coalitions as well as developing a step-wise conservative and surgical approach for their treatment can alleviate patient
symptomatology and provide excellent long-term benefits. Conservative
treatment consists of immobilization, NSAIDs, and casting for symptomatic patients, and surgical treatment for symptomatic tarsal coalition consists of resection and/or arthrodesis.

Lucian M. Feraru and Mark E. Solomon

Pediatric equinus is broadly defined as generalized limited dorsiflexion at
the ankle joint. It may result from either congenital or acquired causes
and exhibit varying characteristics such as flexible, rigid, or spastic types.
It has been extensively studied in literature and is known to be associated
with the pathological condition of the bone, soft tissue, or combined deformity. In children, rigid plantarflexed cases can be debilitating and prevent
them from ambulating without pain, if at all. As this volume in Clinics has
chapters on comprehensive pediatric examination and neuromuscular disorders, this article will focus on (non-neurologic equinus) and its treatment
via conservative and surgical methods with an emphasis on gradual
correction.

# CLINICS IN PODIATRIC MEDICINE AND SURGERY

**SERIES OF RELATED INTEREST**

*Orthopedic Clinics*
https://www.orthopedic.theclinics.com/
*Clinics in Sports Medicine*
https://www.sportsmed.theclinics.com/
*Foot and Ankle Clinics*
https://www.foot.theclinics.com/
*Physical Medicine and Rehabilitation Clinics*
https://www.pmr.theclinics.com/

**THE CLINICS ARE AVAILABLE ONLINE!**
Access your subscription at:
www.theclinics.com

# Foreword

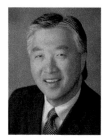

Thomas J. Chang, DPM
*Consulting Editor*

The topic of Pediatric Orthopedics has never been covered in *Clinics in Podiatric Medicine and Surgery*. Why not? Although the profession has been treating pediatric patients from the very beginning, the subspecialty of Podopediatric Medicine is gaining more excitement over the past decade. Within *Clinics in Podiatric Medicine and Surgery*, there have been two publications in the past: Pediatric Foot Deformities, which came out in 2013, and Pediatric Pes Planovalgus, which came out in 2010. There have been several societies focused on the dissemination of podopediatric education. The American College of Podo-pediatrics started within the American Podiatric Medical Association in the 1970s, and currently, membership is growing within the American College of Foot and Ankle Pediatrics, under the guidance of Dr Louis DeCaro.

Pioneers of podopodiatric medicine deserve mention. We are grateful for the vision of Drs James Ganley, Ed Harris, Richard Jay, Russell Volpe, Gary Dockery, Don Green, and Steve Smith. Many have also learned personally from Ignacio Ponseti, MD, who has changed the way the world approaches the newborn clubfoot deformity. I have also been impressed with the current teachings and passion in this area from Drs Patrick Deheer, Patrick Agnew, and Mitzi Williams.

I am also impressed with the growing number of international medical mission trips and the wonderful organizations dedicated to providing state-of-the-art surgical and nonsurgical care to children throughout the world. Special recognition goes out to Healing the Children, Baja Crippled Children's Project, Podiatry Institute Medical Missions, Yucatan Crippled Children's Project, KP Global Health, WorldWalk, and Steps2Walk. This is by no means an exclusive list.

As a father of 3 kids, I have found that there is rarely anything more valuable to me than their health. Consumers of health care often will research specialty care for their children more diligently than they will for themselves. It is prudent for us to continue our education within this topic and be well versed in serving our patients confidently. I applaud Dr Mark Solomon for his efforts in providing this invaluable knowledge to

Clin Podiatr Med Surg 39 (2022) ix–x
https://doi.org/10.1016/j.cpm.2021.11.001
0891-8422/21/© 2021 Published by Elsevier Inc.

the foot and ankle community. I am hopeful this area of Podiatric Medicine will continue to gain momentum in the years to come.

Thomas J. Chang, DPM
Redwood Orthopedic Surgery Associates
208 Concourse Boulevard
Santa Rosa, CA 95403, USA

*E-mail address:*
thomaschang14@comcast.net

# Clubfoot

Mark A. Rieger, MD[a],*, Matthew B. Dobbs, MD[b]

KEYWORDS

- Clubfoot • Clubfeet • Talipes equinovarus • Ponseti • Review article
- Anterior tibial tendon transfer

KEY POINTS

- The Ponseti method is the gold standard of treatment for both idiopathic and nonidiopathic clubfoot and should be initiated as early as possible.
- Brace wear after correction if maintained until age 4 decreases the risk of relapse and increases foot mobility.
- Relapse in children less than 3 years old should initially be treated with recasting followed by bracing.
- Relapse after age 3 requires casting and anterior tibialis transfer and possible Achilles tenotomy.
- Resistant clubfoot needs to be addressed with an a la carte approach.

 Video content accompanies this article at http://www.podiatric.theclinics.com.

## INTRODUCTION

Talipes equinovarus, also referred to as clubfoot, is one of the most common musculoskeletal congenital anomalies. Clubfoot occurs in 0.39 to 7 per 1000 newborns across ethnic populations.[1–4] It is unilateral in 50% of the cases, with the right side being dominant.[5] There are 4 elements of clubfeet: equinus positioning of the hindfoot, varus positioning of the calcaneus, a cavus arch, and metatarsus adductus (**Fig. 1**). This positioning is related to the Achilles tendon being contracted, with a severe shortening of the deltoid and spring ligament in conjunction with tightness of the tibialis posterior and medial tarsal ligaments. This causes the navicular and cuboid to be medially displaced and inverted and the calcaneus to be adducted under the talus creating heel varus. The heel varus combined with the navicular and cuboid inversion and adduction causes the foot to assume a supinated position. The increased flexion of the first metatarsal relative to the lateral metatarsals creates a cavus deformity.[6]

[a] The Pediatric Orthopedic Center, Cedar Knolls, NJ 07927, USA; [b] Dobbs Clubfoot Center, Paley Orthopaedic and Spine Institute, West Palm Beach, FL 33404, USA
* Corresponding author.
E-mail address: Mark.Rieger@consensushealth.com

Clin Podiatr Med Surg 39 (2022) 1–14
https://doi.org/10.1016/j.cpm.2021.08.006
0891-8422/22/© 2021 Elsevier Inc. All rights reserved.

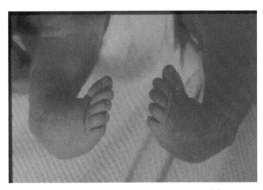

**Fig. 1.** Clubfoot with equinus, varus cavus, and metatarsus adductus.

The common goal of treatment throughout the ages has been to correct these deformities and obtain a foot that is normal in appearance, function, mobility and is pain free. Manipulation, surgical interventions, and combination of manipulation and surgical intervention have been described to attain this goal. Idiopathic or isolated clubfoot is the most common form; however, clubfoot is also seen with a host of neuromuscular disorders, including myelomeningocele, arthrogryposis, static encephalopathy, polio as well as with several genetic syndromes. Isolated clubfoot is familial in as many as 20% of patients. Several genes have been implicated to date for familial clubfoot. It is the goal of this article to briefly review the history of the treatments for clubfoot, discuss its pathogenesis and classification systems, describe treatments that have provided the most successful outcomes, and review complications of treatment and relapse and ways to avoid them.

## HISTORY

Clubfoot has been known to exist since the twelfth century BC when it was noted on the mummy of Egyptian pharaoh Siptah.[7] It was also described in ancient times with the Greek God Hephaestus, who was painted with a congenitally deformed foot.[8,9] The first attempted treatment of clubfoot was described by Hippocrates of Kos in 400 BC. He expressed that treatment should be initiated early and described a method of repeated manipulation followed by the application of strong bandages to obtain foot correction. He further suggested that the corrected foot should be maintained by wearing special shoes.[10] There was no significant change in this treatment until the eighteenth century when tenotomy was introduced as a treatment for clubfoot.[11,12] Aggressive manipulation of the foot and surgical options were expanded in the nineteenth century with the discovery of anesthesia (1846), the introduction of antiseptic technique (1867), and the Esmarch bandage (1873) that minimized blood loss.[13] Devices such as the Thomas wrench were used to forcibly manipulate the foot, and the correction was maintained with plaster of Paris bandages. However, this technique generally left the patient with a stiff, painful, and often still deformed foot.[13] Surgical soft tissue procedures initiated by Phelps in the York in 1881[14] were expanded on by Elmslie,[15] along with bony procedures described by Ogston[16] during this period. Soft tissue surgical procedures prevailed, and more extensive procedures as described by Turco, McKay, and Simons were developed.[17–23] Long term, these extensive surgical soft tissue releases led to poor foot function.[24,25] Concurrently during the period that operative techniques were being expanded, nonoperative approaches were pursued, the most common method by Kite, who in 1939 described a manipulation and serial casting technique.[26,27] This technique however required soft tissue surgical releases in 50% to 75% of the cases in order to obtain full correction.[28] The high nonsurgical failure rate was due to abduction of the foot at the midtarsal joints and applying direct pressure on the calcaneocuboid joint. This maneuver blocked the calcaneus from adducting under the talus, leading to persistent heel varus.

The Ponseti technique (**Fig. 2**) was based on the Farabeuf publication of 1872,[29] which described how the calcaneus rotates under the talus, and adduction, flexion, and inversion occur with a normal foot. This provided the foundation for Ponseti to develop his technique in which he published his first long-term results in 1963,[30] which overcame the obstacles of the Kite technique based on Farabeuf's work. The Ponseti technique now has become the standard of care throughout the world.[31] The Ponseti technique ultimately combines the best of both approaches with its emphasis on soft tissue manipulation and minimal surgical intervention in the form of a percutaneous tenotomy and maintenance with a brace.

## CAUSE

The most common form of clubfoot is idiopathic/isolated.[5] Clubfoot is also found in association with a host of neuromuscular disorders, including myelodysplasia, arthrogryposis as well as with several known genetic syndromes, including but not limited to arthrogryposis, Down syndrome, diastrophic dysplasia, and Larsen syndrome. Environmental factors also likely play a role in clubfoot. Early amniocentesis during the first trimester, maternal smoking, exposure to viral infection, maternal diabetes, and maternal age have all been reported to be risk factors for clubfoot.[5,32–34]

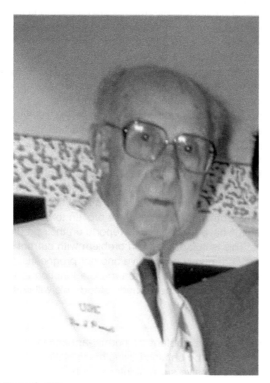

**Fig. 2.** Ignacio V. Ponseti, MD.

## EVALUATION AND CLASSIFICATION

There are 4 types of clubfoot described, which are based on cause: (1) postural, (2) idiopathic, (3) neurogenic, and (4) syndromic. Postural clubfoot generally can be stretched and occasionally casted; this is the definitive form of treatment. Idiopathic clubfoot has no known cause but has rigid components and generally will require casting, Achilles tendon tenotomy, and maintenance of position for several years. Many within this category are familial and have a genetic cause, but a formal classification system has yet to be developed to more accurately describe this group. The type of clubfoot within this group is heterogeneous with some responding well to casting and others that are more difficult. Genetics is the key to explaining this difference to responsiveness to treatment and is based on more severe lack of development of muscle in the lower limb in resistant patients. On occasion, more extensive surgery will be required and has significant risk of relapse. Neurogenic clubfoot is associated with underlying neurologic conditions, such as myelomeningocele, and last, there is a syndromic clubfoot, which is generally rigid and can be associated with anomalies.[35] Ponseti and colleagues[36] have also reported what they call a complex idiopathic clubfoot that was defined as having rigid equinus, severe plantar flexion of all metatarsals, a deep crease above the heel, a transverse crease in the sole of the foot, and the shortened hyperextended first toe. These features are not seen at birth but develop during the casting process and often are seen after cast slipping.

Over the years, there have been many classification systems to assess the severity of idiopathic clubfoot based on physical aspects of the foot.[37–46] The 2 systems now used commonly are the Pirani score[45] and Dimegleo scale[41] classifications. The Dimeglio classifies a clubfoot into 4 types: grade I to grade IV. A lower grade represents a less severe deformity. The following parameters are evaluated in the sagittal and horizontal plane. Sagittal plane measurements evaluated are equinus and varus rotation. Horizontal plane measurements are evaluated for derotation and forefoot adduction relative to the hindfoot. Each item receives a score of 0 to 4 points with a maximum of 20 points. Using these parameters, the foot is graded I to IV. Grade I, benign, is reducible without any resistance; grade II to grade III, moderate and severe, are reducible against resistance, and type 4, severe, is not reducible.

The Pirani scoring system was designed to assess the severity and progress of treatment using the Ponseti method. The system is based on the physical appearance of the foot. There are 3 morphologic signs in the hindfoot: posterior crease, emptiness of the heel, and rigid equinus. There are an additional 3 morphologic signs in the midfoot: lateral curvature of the foot, medial crease, position of the head of the talus on the lateral border. Each one of these 6 parameters are graded as 0, normal; 0.5, mildly abnormal; 1, severe abnormal, and there can be a total score of 6, with 6 being the most severe deformity. Both classifications have proven to be very reproducible.[47,48] However, these systems have had equivocal reports on their predictiveness in treatment outcomes.[49–53] This is in fact the main problem with current classification systems for clubfoot: they are purely descriptive and not prognostic. What is needed is a classification system that is based also on muscle function in the lower limb. As the genetic aspects of clubfoot are better understood, this will come to fruition.

## TREATMENT

The end result for treatment of a clubfoot is a normal-appearing foot that is mobile and pain free. These goals should be obtained using manipulation of the soft tissues and avoiding when possible extensive surgical intervention. The 2 techniques that have been shown to obtain this goal are the Ponseti method and the French method. The

French method requires daily manipulation of the newborn clubfoot by a skilled physiotherapist. The correction is maintained with taping of the foot and ankle. To maintain motion, a continuous passive motion machine is also instituted. The French technique requires daily treatments for 2 months and then decreases to 3 times a week until 6 months of age and is maintained by the parents performing the stretching daily. After correction, the child's feet are maintained in Denis Brown bar and shoes. The success rate for this technique has been reported by Dimeglio in 1990 to be 74% successful.[54] There are other studies that suggest a lower success rate,[55,56] yet others that have found it comparable to the Ponseti technique.[55] There is a higher reported need for later posterior soft tissue release in patients treated with the French method, as the equinus does not respond well to manipulation alone in many patients with clubfoot. Because of the intensity of this technique and higher surgical rate, the French method has fallen out of favor, and the Ponseti technique remains the main form of treatment throughout the world. However, the use of stretching as part of the maintenance of clubfoot correction after initial correction with Ponseti casting is a hybrid model that makes sense.

The Ponseti method used to correct clubfoot was developed by Ignacio Ponseti in the 1940s at the University of Iowa medical school. Ponseti describes in his article, Congenital clubfoot fundamental of treatment,[6] that during his training he observed multiple forms of nonoperative attempts at correcting clubfoot, most of which ended up with surgical correction. Ponseti himself expanded the medial release operation to include a posterior release and often made a lateral incision to free the tarsal joints to align the tarsal bones with the cuneiform to metatarsals. He realized the surgery left deep scarring, joint stiffness, and weakness. He observed Kite, who at the time was the leading advocate of conservative treatment, and ultimately came to the conclusion that the failure of treatment of clubfoot related to poor understanding of the fundamental anatomy of the normal foot and the clubfoot. He studied the pathologic changes of the clubfoot and came to understand that the fundamental mistake that Kite was making was applying pressure to the calcaneocuboid joint and not releasing the subtalar joint first. Ponseti, understanding the physiology of the clubfoot, realized by placing pressure on the first metatarsal and supinating the foot he could unlock the calcaneus and talus, which is now understood to be essential as the initial step in the corrective manipulation of a clubfoot. This was the beginning of the Ponseti method that has revolutionized the treatment of clubfoot.

The Ponseti method involves serial manipulation of the foot, which is then maintained by a long leg cast (**Fig. 3**). The manipulations are performed in a specific manner to achieve correction of the 4 elements of equinovarus foot. With the exception of the cavus deformity, which is corrected as the first step with a supination maneuver, the rest of the deformities are then corrected simultaneously with external rotation of the foot using the head of the talus as the fulcrum (Video 1). Although equinus of the subtalar complex does correct some with external rotation of the foot, it usually does not

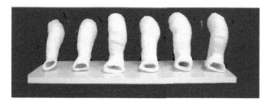

**Fig. 3.** Serial Ponseti casts.

correct enough. Therefore, most patients require an Achilles tendon tenotomy to achieve full correction[57] **(Fig. 4)**. Once the tenotomy is performed, a final Ponseti cast is applied **(Fig. 5)** and is removed after 3 weeks. Once correction is obtained **(Fig. 6)**, it needs to be maintained by a foot abduction orthosis for a prolonged period to minimize the risk of relapses **(Fig. 7)**. It also provides for different strategies to treat relapses, which are based on the patient's age at the time of relapse. Successful treatment involves multiple foot manipulation maintained by casting, Achilles tendon tenotomy, and nighttime bracing in most patients until the age of 4 years. It cannot be overemphasized the importance of communicating with the family from the onset of treatment what is involved and the importance of their commitment to the successful outcome of treatment.

Ideally, serial casting should commence as soon after birth as possible. The casting will consist of gentle foot manipulations, which are performed in an office setting followed by serial application of long leg cast as described by Ponseti.[31,57] Short leg casts are to be avoided because of a higher failure rate.[58] Plaster casting was the original method described by Ponseti; however, fiberglass material has been demonstrated to be effective in some hands.[31,59] Casting is changed either twice a week or once a week depending on the use of a standard or accelerated protocol,[60–62] and good results have been reported with either method. The accelerated protocol is best used in patients less than 12 months of age, as after 1 year of age leaving casts on for a week at a time gives a more effective stretch. Both protocols require an average of 5 casts, so with the accelerated protocol, children are in a cast half as long as the standard.

The initial steps of the Ponseti technique are critical. Cavus deformities are corrected first by supinating the forefoot with direct pressure under the first metatarsal. A long-leg cast is applied in 2 stages. First, a short-leg cast is completed; then the knee is flexed to 90°, and the cast is extended into a long-leg cast. Generally, the cavus deformity is corrected with a single cast. Next, the hindfoot varus, forefoot adduction, and hindfoot equinus are simultaneously corrected with the next 3 to 4 casts. This is done by gently abducting the foot in supination while counterpressure is applied to the head of the talus. It is imperative to note that the fulcrum point laterally is the talar head and not the calcaneocuboid joint, which is used with Kite's technique. After this set of casts is completed, all deformities are usually corrected except for the hindfoot equinus. The foot should be able to be abducted to 50°, and hindfoot varus should be corrected. Once this has been achieved, tenotomy of the Achilles tendon is

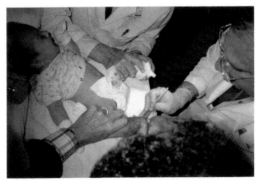

**Fig. 4.** In-office tenotomy.

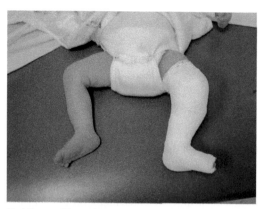

**Fig. 5.** Properly applied Ponseti long leg cast.

performed to correct the equinus contracture. It is generally accepted that approximately 90% of cases requires tenotomy.

In children less than 1 year of age, a tenotomy can be performed with topical local anesthetic and posttenotomy injection of an anesthetic. Injection of anesthetic should be avoided before tenotomy, as it obscures the anatomy and increases risk of injury to the neurovascular bundle.[63] If a child is greater than 1 year of age, formal sedation in an operating room is recommended to control the environment when performing the tenotomy. It is important to note that the tendon is not lengthened; rather, a formal transection of the tendon is the goal of the tenotomy. Once the Achilles tendon is

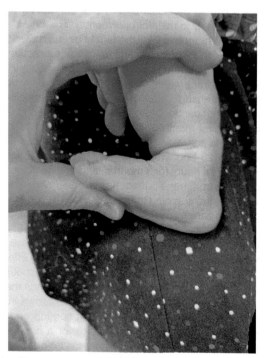

**Fig. 6.** Foot 3 weeks after tenotomy with full dorsiflexion and intact Achilles tendon.

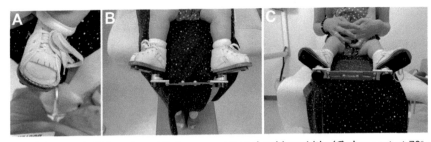

**Fig. 7.** (A) Properly fitting shoe; (B) shoes are set at shoulder width; (C) shoes set at 70° of external rotation.

transected, a sterile dressing is applied, and a final long-leg cast is placed with the foot position at 70° of abduction if possible and 5° to 10° of dorsiflexion. It should be noted that all clubfeet will achieve 70° of abduction. Complex clubfeet, for instance, should not be abducted greater than 50° nor should clubfeet be associated with arthrogryposis or other neurogenic disorders. Attempts to do so in more rigid feet can result in midfoot break. This cast is left on for 3 weeks after tenotomy at which time the tendon should be healed.[64–66] It is generally accepted that the Achilles tenotomy can be performed up to 2 years of age.

After the final cast is removed, the patient is immediately placed in a foot abduction brace. The brace is worn 23 hours a day for 3 months. The shoe is set on the bar to the final degree of external rotation achieved in the last cast for a clubfoot and 30° for a non-clubfoot. If the orthotist is instructed to set all clubfeet at 70°, there will be a high incidence of brace intolerance. If only 50° of external rotation was achieved in the last cast, the brace should be set at 50°. The brace cannot be used to achieve correction; it can only be used to maintain correction. The bar is set to the width of the child's shoulders. It is imperative that the family be instructed in proper donning and doffing of the shoes. Too loose can result in loss of correction or slipping out of the brace and sores on the feet and heels. Too tight can result in sores developing on the foot and heel and brace intolerance. It is important to be available to talk with the family early on to ensure bracing is going well. Patients are seen again if they are having problems that cannot be solved on the telephone or online. Otherwise, returning at the end of the first month is appropriate, then 2 months later, and then at 3-month intervals during the first year of bracing. Bracing hours are gradually weaned after the initial 3 months of 23-hour wear to ensure tolerance. Eighteen hours is used for the next 3 months, then 14 hours for 3 months, and then night and naptime until the fourth birthday in most children. If the patient has experienced relapses or has weakness in the lower extremity, then bracing time is extended beyond the age of 4 years. It must be emphasized to the parents the importance of compliance with this program to minimize the risk of relapse.

There are many different styles of abduction foot braces that are available to maintain foot correction. The author has found although they all are effective, children are sometimes more adaptable to a particular style of brace, and it should be expressed to the family that a brace style may need to be changed to enhance the patient's compliance with bracing. One brace that has a dynamic bar that allows independent movement of each leg has the potential to improve patient comfort and improves bracing tolerance.[67–69] Ankle foot orthosis cannot substitute for a bar and shoes because they have been shown to have a significantly higher failure rate.[70,71] Children braced greater than 36 months have better mobility than those who were not.[72,73]

The Ponseti method is now applied globally and is considered the method of choice in the treatment of clubfoot since 2000.[74] With increasing experience and success, the indications have expanded to treat children older than 1 year old with neglected club-foot with satisfactory outcomes (89%) and low recurrence rate (18%)[49,75–77] and has now been used successfully with more severe nonidiopathic clubfoot deformities. The technique has been applied to arthrogryposis,[67,78,79] meningocele,[80–82] multiple ge-netic syndromes,[69] and neuromuscular disorders.[67,69] Success rate as reported in a systematic review article of nonidiopathic clubfoot demonstrated an initial correction rate of 92% in both idiopathic and nonidiopathic clubfeet, and both groups required approximately 7 casts. Recurrence rate was 11% in idiopathic, whereas recurrence rate in nonidiopathic clubfeet was 43%. The idiopathic clubfeet had a 95% overall successful outcome compared with 69% successful outcome for the nonidiopathic clubfeet.[83] The Ponseti method has also been adapted to the complex idiopathic clubfoot.[36]

Despite the success with the Ponseti method, clubfoot relapse continues to be an issue when treating a clubfoot. It occurs in approximately 1 in 3 clubfoot patients, with a range of 3.7% to 67% that correlated with the mean duration of the study follow-up. The relapse rate also decreased with increasing age.[72,84] The risk factors for recur-rence is associated with the severity of the deformity,[85] the quality of muscle develop-ment in the lower limb, and poor compliance with bracing.[86] Most early-occurring relapses can be treated with repeat casting followed by reapplication of a foot abduc-tion brace. If casting is unable to obtain 15° of dorsiflexion, then the tenotomy needs to be repeated. If a child is 3 years old or older with a varus hindfoot and a dynamic su-pination of the forefoot while ambulating, then the varus hindfoot and adduction of the foot are corrected with serial casting. It is important to ensure full reduction of the anteroposterior talocalcaneal angle with casting. Residual subluxation will result in recurrent deformity. Then, a full tibialis anterior tendon transfer to the third cuneiform is performed. At the same time, any residual equinus should be corrected. The child is casted for 6 weeks and then referred to physical therapy for muscle strengthening and gait training. A nighttime stretching splint is used for a year on average, and daytime splinting is used for around 6 weeks. This procedure has been shown to efficiently cor-rect recurrent dynamic deformity.[87] Other procedures may need to be performed on an a la carte basis and include cuboid-cuneiform osteotomy, posterior ankle and sub-talar release, heel cord tenotomy and plantar fascia release, and rarely, comprehen-sive posteromedial release or correction by gradual distraction.[88,89] Formal physical therapy can be a useful adjunct to prevent relapse in patients with documented weak-ness in the lower legs. Patients with weak foot evertors are particularly prone to relapse and benefit from early and aggressive physical therapy.

## DISCUSSION

Clubfoot is one of the most common musculoskeletal anomalies affecting the lower extremity. The purpose of this review was to provide a prospective on the history of clubfoot treatment and how it led to the present gold standard of treatment, which is the Ponseti method. Because of the success of the Ponseti method, it has been applied to children greater than 1 year of age and nonidiopathic clubfeet. Despite its high initial success rate, there are many reports of relapse. Various treatment op-tions to treat relapse and obtain a pain-free, dynamically mobile foot that is maintained long term have been proposed. Review of the literature demonstrates that the Ponseti technique can be reinstituted to regain correction of a recurrent clubfoot up to age 3 years. After age 3, an anterior tibialis tendon transfer supplemented on occasion with an Achilles tendon tenotomy can obtain this goal. With nonidiopathic clubfoot, which generally is more resistant to treatment, and the more severe clubfoot treated with the Ponseti technique, relapse is treated similarly as idiopathic, but other options may have to be considered on an a la carte basis.

## SUMMARY

Equinovarus deformity is the most common congenital anomaly affecting the lower extremities. The cause of isolated clubfoot is heterogeneous, but genetic factors clearly play a role in many patients. There are 2 well-established classification systems, Pirani and Dimeglio, which can be useful to judge progress in a patient's treatment. The goal of treatment is to obtain a normal-appearing foot that is mobile and pain free and lasts long term without any extensive soft tissue release. The best technique to achieve this goal is with manipulation using the Ponseti technique and supplemented by an Achilles tendon tenotomy in most patients. This technique generally obtains an excellent result; however, this must be maintained with the use of foot abduction bracing at nighttime for a minimum of 2 years. However, the long-term results tend to be better maintained if bracing is extended for 4 years. Stretching exercises for the clubfoot can be taught to all parents and are a good way to engage parents in the treatment protocol and to improve motion in the foot and ankle during the bracing stage. The most common treatment option for relapse initially is recasting. If that is not effective, then anterior tibialis tendon transfer should strongly be considered with other possible soft tissue procedures.

## CLINICS CARE POINTS

- Understanding the clubfoot physiology is essential in treat of clubfoot.
- Plantar pressure on the first metatarsal and foot supination unlocks the calcaneus and talus and is the essential first step to the Ponseti technique.
- Hindfoot varus, forefoot adduction and hindfoot equinus are simultaneously corrected by abduction the the forefoot in supination while counter pressure is applied to the talar head.
- Long term bracing after correction correlates with a decrease in relapse.

## DISCLOSURE

M.A. Rieger and M.B. Dobbs: No disclosures.

## SUPPLEMENTARY DATA

Supplementary data related to this article can be found online at https://doi.org/10.1016/j.cpm.2021.08.006.

## REFERENCES

1. Wynne-Davies R. Genetic and environmental factors in the etiology of talipes equinovarus. Clin Orthop Relat Res 1972;84:9–13.
2. Beals RK. Club foot in the Maori: a genetic study of 50 kindreds. N Z Med J 1978; 88:144–6.
3. Chung CS, Nemechek RW, Larsen IJ, et al. Genetic and epidemiological studies of clubfoot in Hawaii. General and medical considerations. Hum Hered 1969;19: 321–42.

4. Dobbs MB, Gurnett CA. Genetics in clubfoot. J Pediatr Orthop 2012;B21(1):7–9.
5. Wynne-Davies R. Family studies and the cause of congenital club foot. J Bone Joint Surg Br 1964;46B:445–63.
6. Ponseti I. Congenital clubfoot essential of treatment. Oxford, England: Oxford University Press; 1996. p. 37–48.
7. Smith EG, Warren RD. Egyptian mummies. London: Allen and Umwin; 1924.
8. Partsocas CS. Hephaestus and clubfoot. Hist Med Allied Sci 1972;27:450–1.
9. Hippocrates and Adams F. The genuine works of Hippocrates. Baltimore, MD: Williams and Wilkins: 1039. pp 21-22
10. Fitzgerald R. Homer use odyssey. New York: Garden City Publishers; 1930. p. 144–9.
11. Hernigou P, Huys M, Pariet J, et al. History of clubfoot treatment, Part 1: from manipulation in antiquity to splint and plaster in Renaissance before tenotomy. Int Orthopaedics (Sicot) 2017;41:1693–704.
12. Sanzarello I, Nanni M, Faldini C. The clubfoot over the centuries. J Pediatr Orthop B 2017;26:143–51.
13. Hernigou P. History of clubfoot treatment, part III (twentieth century): back to the future. Int Orthop 2017;41:2407–14.
14. Phelps AM. A case of double talipes equinovarus treated by open incision and fixed extension. New Engl Mon 1881;11:195.
15. Elmslie RC. The principles of treatment of congenital talipes equinovarus. J Orthop Surg 1920;2:669.
16. Ogston A. A new principle of curing club-foot in severe cases in children a few years old. Br Med J 1902;1:1524–6.
17. Turco VJ. Surgical correction of the resistant club foot. J Bone Joint Surg Am 1971;53:477–97.
18. McKay DW. New concept of and approach to clubfoot treatment: section I – principles and morbid anatomy. J Pediatr Orthop 1982;2:347–56.
19. McKay DW. New concept of an approach to clubfoot treatment: section II – correction of the clubfoot. J Pediatr Orthop 1983;3:10–21.
20. McKay DW. New concept of and approach to clubfoot treatment: section III- evaluation and results. J Pediatr Orthop 1983;3:141–8.
21. Simons GW. Complete subtalar release in club feet. Part I – a preliminary report. J Bone Joint Surg Am 1985;67:1044–55.
22. Simons GW. Complete subtalar release in club feet. Part II—comparison with less extensive procedures 1985;67:1056–65.
23. Simons GW. Surgical correction of clubfeet. Oper Tech Orthop 1993;3:103–14.
24. Cooper DM, Dietz FR. Treatment of idiopathic clubfoot. A thirty-year follow-up note. J Bone Joint Surg Am 1995;77:1477–89.
25. Dobbs MB, Nunley R, Schoenecker PL. Long-term follow-up of patients with clubfeet treated with extensive soft-tissue release. J Bone Joint Surg Am 2006;88: 986–96.
26. Kite JH. Some suggestions on the treatment of club foot by casts. J Bone Joint Surg Am 1963;45:406–12.
27. Kite JH. Principles involved in the treatment of congenital club-foot. 1939. J Bone Joint Surg Am 2003;85:1847.
28. Lovell WW, Farley D. Treatment of congenital clubfoot. ONA J 1979;6:453–6.
29. Farabeuf LH. Pricis de manual operative. 4th edition. Paris: Masson; 1983.
30. Ponseti IV, Smoley EN. Congenital clubfoot: the results of treatment. J Bone Joint Surg Am 1963;45:261–344.

31. Ponseti IV. Treatment of congenital club foot. J Bone Joint Surg Am 1992;74: 448–54.
32. Foster A, Davis N. Congenital talipes equinovarus (clubfoot) surgery 2007;25(4): 171–5.
33. Siapkara A, Duncan R. Congenital talipes equinovarus: a review of current management. J Bone Joint Surg Br 2007;89(8):995–1000.
34. Gibbons PJ, Gray K. Update on clubfoot. J Paediatr Child Health 2013;49(3): E434–7.
35. Balasankar G, Luximon A, Al-Jumaily A. Current conservative management and classification of club foot: a review. J Pediatr Rehab Med 2016;9:257–64.
36. Ponseti IV, Shivkov M, Davis N. Treatment of the complex idiopathic clubfoot. Clin Orthop Rel Res 2006;451:171–6.
37. Cummings RJ, Davidson RS, Armstrong PF, et al. Congenital clubfoot. J Bone Joint Surg Am 2002;84:290–308.
38. Harrold AJ, Walker CJ. Treatment and prognosis in congenital clubfoot. J Bone Joint Surg Br 1983;65:8–11.
39. Ponseti IV, Smoley EN. The classic: congenital club foot: the results of treatment 1963. Clin Orthop Relat Res 2009;467:1133–45.
40. Catterall A. A method of assessment of the clubfoot deformity. Clin Orthop Relat Res 1991;264:48–53.
41. Dimeglio A, Bensahel H, Souchet P, et al. Classification of clubfoot. J Pediatr Orthop B 1995;4:129–36.
42. Carroll NC. Preoperative clinical evaluation of clubfoot. In: Simons GW, editor. The clubfoot: the present and a view of the future. New York: Springer-Verlag; 1994. p. 97–8.
43. Goldner JL, Fitch RD. Classification and evaluation of congenital talipes equinovarus. In: Simons GW, editor. The clubfoot: the present and a view of the future. New York: Springer-Verlag; 1994. p. 120–39.
44. Pandey S, Pandey AK. Clinical classification of congenital clubfeet. In: Simons GW, editor. The clubfoot: the present and a view of the future. New York: Springer-Verlag; 1994. p. 91–2.
45. Pirani S, Outerbridge HK, Sawatzky B, et al. A reliable method of clinically evaluating a virgin clubfoot evaluation. 21st SICOT Congress. Sydney, Australia, April 18-23, 1999.
46. Stevens D, Meyer S. CTEV equinus severity grading scale. In: Simons GW, editor. The clubfoot: the present and a view of the future. New York: Springer-Verlag; 1994. p. 98–102.
47. Flynn JM, Donohoe M, Mackenzie WG. An independent assessment of two clubfoot-classification systems. J Pediatr Orthop 1998;18:323–7.
48. Cosma D, VAsilescu DE. A clinical evaluation of the Pirani and Dimeglio idiopathic clubfoot classification. J Foot Ankle Surg 2015;54:582–5.
49. Dobbs MB, Rudzki JR, Purcell DB, et al. Factors predictive of outcome after use of the Ponseti method for the treatment of idiopathic clubfeet. J Bone Joint Surg Am 2004;86:22–7.
50. Crawford HA. Early clubfoot recurrence after use of the Ponseti method in a New Zealand population. J Bone Joint Surg Am 2007;89:487–93.
51. Dyer PJ, Davis N. The role of the Pirani scoring system in the management of clubfoot by the Ponseti method. J Bone Joint Surg Br 2006;88:1082–4.
52. Scher DM, Feldman DS, van Bosse HJP, et al. Predicting the need for tenotomy in the Ponseti method for correction of clubfeet. J Pediatr Orthop 2004;24:349–52.

53. Chu A, Labar BS, Sala DA, et al. Clubfoot classification: correlation with Ponseti cast treatment. J Pediatr Orthop 2010;30:695–9.

54. Bensahel H, Catterall A, Dimeglio A. Practical applications in idiopathic clubfoot: a retrospective multicentric study in EPOS. J Pediatr Orthop 1990;10:186–8.

55. Richards BS, Faulks S, Rathjen KE, et al. A comparison of two nonoperative methods of idiopathic clubfoot correction: the Ponseti method and the French functional (physiotherapy) method. J Bone Joint Surg Am 2008;90:2313–21.

56. Campenhout A, Molenaers G, Moens P, et al. Does functional treatment of idiopathic clubfoot reduce the indication for surgery? Call for a widely accepted rating system. J Pediatr Orthop B 2001;10:315–8.

57. Laaveg SJ, Ponseti IV. Long-term results of treatment of congenital club foot. J Bone Joint Surg Am 1980;62:23–31.

58. Maripuri SN, Gallacher PD, Bridgens J, et al. Ponseti casting for club foot – above – or below-knee?: a prospective randomized clinical trial. Bone Joint J 2013;95-B: 1570–4.

59. Pittner DE, Klingele KE, Beebe AC. Treatment of clubfoot with the Ponseti method: a comparison of casting materials. J Pediatr Orthop 2008;28:250–3.

60. Morcuende JA, Abbasi D, Dolan LA, et al. Results of an accelerated Ponseti protocol for clubfoot. J Pediatr Orthop 2005;25:623–6.

61. Islam MS, Masood QM, Bashir A, et al. Results of a standard versus an accelerated Ponseti protocol for clubfoot: a prospective randomized study. Clin Orthop Surg 2020;12(1):100–6.

62. Elgohary HS, Abulsaad M. Traditional and accelerated Ponseti technique: a comparative study. Eur J Orthop Surg Traumatol 2015;25(5):949–53.

63. Dobbs MB, Gordon JE, Walton T, et al. Bleeding complications following percutaneous tendoachilles tenotomy in the treatment of clubfoot deformity. J Pediatr Orthop 2004;24:353–7.

64. Saini R, Dhillon MS, Tripathy SK, et al. Regeneration of the Achilles tendon after percutaneous tenotomy in infants: a clinical and MRI study. J Pediatr Orthop B 2010;19:344–7.

65. Mangatht KS, Kanwar R, Johnson K, et al. Ultrasonographic phases in gap healing following Ponseti-type Achilles tenotomy. J Bone Joint Surg Am 2010;92:1462–7.

66. Niki H, Nakajima H, Hirano T, et al. Ultrasonographic observation of the healing process in the gap after a Ponseti-type Achilles tenotomy for idiopathic congenital clubfoot at two-year follow-up. J Orthop Sci 2012;18:70–5.

67. Boehm S, Limpaphayom N, Alaee F, et al. Early results of the Ponseti method for the treatment of clubfoot in distal arthrogryposis. J Bone Joint Surg Am 2008;90:1501–7.

68. Chen RC, Gordon JE, Luhmann SJ, et al. A new dynamic foot abduction orthosis for clubfoot treatment. J Pediatr Orthop 2007;27:522–8.

69. Gurnett CA, Boehm S, Connolly A, et al. Impact of congenital talipes equinovarus etiology on treatment outcomes. Dev Med Child Neurol 2008;50:498–502.

70. George HL, Unnikrishnan PN, Garg NK, et al. Unilateral foot abduction orthosis: is it a substitute for Denis Browne boots following Ponseti technique? J Pediatr Orthop B 2010;20:22–5.

71. Janicki JA, Wright JG, Weir S, et al. A comparison of ankle foot orthoses with foot abduction orthoses to prevent recurrence following correction of idiopathic clubfoot by the Ponseti method. J Bone Joint Surg Br 2011;93:700–4.

72. Khan AA, Abarca N, Cung NQ, et al. Use of PROMIS in assessment of children with Ponseti-treated idiopathic clubfoot: better scores with greater than 3 years of brace use. J Pediatr Ortho 2020;40(9):526–30.

73. Agarwal A, Rastogi A, Rastogi P, et al. Relapses in clubfoot treated with Ponseti technique and standard bracing protocol- a systematic analysis. J Clin Orthop Traum 2021;18:199–204.

74. Zionts LE, Ebramzadeh E, Morgan R, et al. Sixty years on: Ponseti method for clubfoot treatment produces high satisfaction despite inherent tendency to relapse. J Bone Joint Surg Am 2018;100:721–8.

75. Lourenco AF, Morcuende JA. Correction of neglected idiopathic club foot by the Ponseti method. J Bone Joint Surg Br 2007;89:378–81.

76. Shah A, Mehta R, Aroojis A. The Ponseti method of clubfoot treatment in walking age children: is it effective? A study of 56 children from 1 to 10 years of age. J Pediatr Orthop B 2019;28(2):159–66.

77. Ferreira GF, Stefani KC, Haje D. The Ponseti method in children with clubfoot after walking age – systematic review and metanalysis of observational studies. PLoS One 2018;13(11):e0207153.

78. Kowalyczyk B, Felus J. Ponseti casting and Achilles release versus classic casting and soft tissue releases for the initial treatment of arthrogrypotic clubfeet. Foot Ankle Int 2015;36:1072–7.

79. Matar HE, Beirne P, Garg N. The effectiveness of the Ponseti method for treating clubfoot associated with arthrogryposis up to 8 years follow-up. J Child Orthop 2016;10:15–8.

80. Janicki JA, Narayanan UG, Havey B, et al. Treatment of neuromuscular and syndrome associated (nonidiopathic) clubfeet using the Ponseti method. J Pediatr Orthop 2009;29:393–7.

81. Gerlach DR, Gurnett A, Limpaphayom N, et al. Early results of the Ponseti method for the treatment of clubfoot associated with myelomeningocele. J Bone Joint Surg Am 2009;91A:1350–9.

82. Matar HE, Veirne P, Garg NK. Effectiveness of the Ponseti method for treating clubfoot associated with myelomeningocele: 3-9 years follow-up. J Pediatr Orthop B 2017;26:133–6.

83. De Mulder T, Prinsen S, Van Campenhout A. Treatment of non-idiopathic clubfeet with the Ponseti method: a systematic review. J Child Orthop 2018;12:575–81.

84. Thomas HM, Sangiorgia SN, Ebramzadeh E, et al. Relapse rates in patients with clubfoot treated using the Ponseti method increase with time a systemic review. JBJS Rev 2019;7(5):1–8.

85. Kuzma AL, Talwalkar VR, Muchow RD, et al. Brace yourselves: outcomes of Ponseti casting and foot abduction orthosis bracing in idiopathic congenital talipes equinovarus. J Pediatr Ortho 2020;40(1):e25–9.

86. Zionts LE, Jew MH, Bauer KL, et al. How many patients who have a clubfoot treated using the Ponseti method are likely to undergo a tendon transfer? J Pediatr Orthop 2018;38(7):382–7.

87. Mindler GT, Kranzl A, Radler C. Normalization of forefoot supination after tibialis anterior tendon transfer for dynamic clubfoot recurrence. J Pediatr Orthop 2020;40(8):418–24.

88. Hosseinzadh P, Kiebzak GM, Dolan L, et al. Management of clubfoot relapses with Ponseti method: results of a survey of the POSNA members. J Pediatr Orthop 2019;39(1):38–41.

89. Hosseinzadh P, Kelly DM, Zionts LE. Management of the relapsed clubfoot following treatment using the Ponseti method. J Am Acad Orthop Surg 2017;25(3):195–203.

# Neurologic Disorders Affecting the Foot and Ankle

William R. Yorns Jr, DO

## KEYWORDS

- Peripheral neuropathy • Ataxia • Nerve entrapment • Cerebral palsy
- Immune-mediated polyneuropathies • Charcot–Marie–Tooth disease

## KEY POINTS

- Hereditary and acquired disorders of foot and leg dysfunction are common in clinical practice.
- A detailed history and examination are essential in determining the etiology and treatment plan.
- Genetic testing is vast and diverse for many of these disorders.

## THE NEUROANATOMY OF THE LEG AND FOOT: OVERVIEW

The focus of this article is to review the neurologic causes and conditions that lead to foot pain, weakness, sensory loss, and/or musculoskeletal deformity. These patients may present to their primary care physician or may also be referred to a podiatrist, neurologist, orthopedics, or physical medicine clinic for consultation. To first understand the neurologic manifestations of foot dysfunction, it will be best to have a brief overview of the nerve distribution in the foot and leg.

The motor and sensory impulses for the foot and leg start in the associated discrete areas of the motor and sensory cortex of the brain. Sensory input from the body follows a dermatologic distribution that coalesces into the sensory nerves that converge into the ventral rootlets of the corresponding vertebral level. These nerves travel into the spinal cord forming, the afferent corticospinal tracts along the ventral service then traveling to the thalamus and lastly to the sensory cortex of the brain (**Fig. 1**). The efferent corticospinal tracts for motor activity start in the primary motor cortex of the brain and travels along the caudal service of the spinal cord through the

Department of Neurology, UCONN School of Medicine, Connecticut Children's Medical Center, 505 Farmington Avenue., 2nd Floor, Farmington, CT 06032, USA
E-mail address: wyorns@connecticutchildrens.org

Clin Podiatr Med Surg 39 (2022) 15–35
https://doi.org/10.1016/j.cpm.2021.08.005     podiatric.theclinics.com

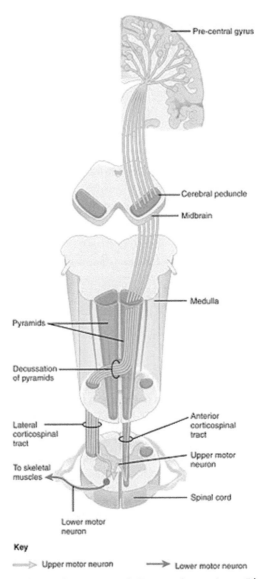

**Fig. 1.** The corticospinal tract. (*From* "Somatic Nervous System Image" by Isa.tomanelli, Wikimedia Commons (https://commons.wikimedia.org/wiki/File:Somatic_Nervous_System_Image.svg) CC BY-SA 4.0.)

corticospinal tracts to synapse on the anterior horn cells and exit the anterior rootlets (**Fig. 2**). Each vertebral level gives rise to an anterior and posterior nerve root that combines to form a mixed (motor and sensory) spinal nerve. These converge in the lower spine to form the lumbar and sacral plexuses of the lower extremity (**Fig. 3**). The 6 large nerves that are formed from the lumbar plexus are the iliohypogastric nerve (L1 with small contribution from T12), ilioinguinal nerve (L1), genitofemoral nerve (L1, L2), lateral femoral cutaneous nerve (L2, L3), obturator nerve (L2, L3, L4), and the femoral nerve

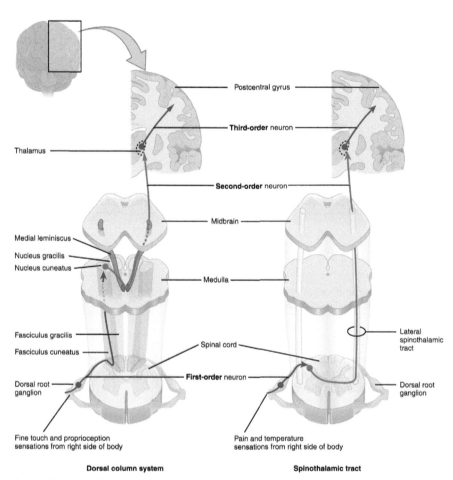

**Fig. 2.** The spinothalamic tract. (*From* 14.2 Central Processing [Image], by Betts, et. al, Anatomy and Physiology, OpenStax College (https://openstax.org/books/anatomy-and-physiology/pages/14-2-central-processing) CC BY 4.0.)

(L2, L3, L4). The sacral plexus arises from vertebral levels L4 to S4 and gives rise to the superior gluteal nerve (L4, L5, S1), inferior gluteal nerve (L5, S1, S2), sciatic nerve (L4, L5, S1), posterior femoral cutaneous nerve (S1, S2, S3), and pudendal nerve (S2, S3, S4). Further smaller divisions off these rami and nerves gives rise to the rest of the nerve innervation of the leg including the cluneal nerves (formed by branches of the rami of L1–S1), genicular nerves (from the sciatic nerve), tibial nerve and common fibular (peroneal) nerve (from the sciatic nerve), saphenous nerve (from the femoral nerve), sural nerve (formed from the tibial and common fibular nerves), superficial and deep fibular nerve (from the common fibular nerve), dorsal digital nerves of the foot (from branches of the sural nerve and deep fibular nerve), plantar digital nerves (from branches off the tibial nerve), lateral dorsal cutaneous nerve (from the sural nerve), and plantar nerves (from the tibial nerve).

The basic knowledge of nerve distribution and innervation gives a framework to further understand the basis of disease for the disorders described in this article.

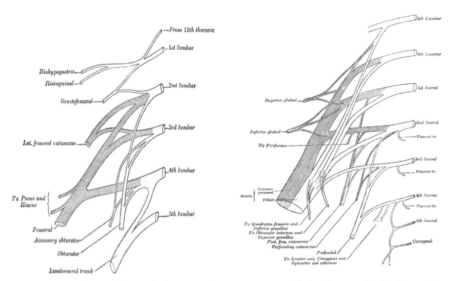

**Fig. 3.** The lumbar and sacral plexuses. (*From* Anatomy of the Human Body (https://en.wikipedia.org/wiki/File:Gray832.png) by Henry Gray, 1918.)

Common disorders of the foot and leg that are associated with neuromuscular conditions are discussed. A review of disease presentation, etiology, signs and symptoms, and diagnostic testing is discussed as well.

## PES CAVUS AND VALGUS

Pes cavus (or cavovarus foot) is a high arched foot that is typically caused by malposition of the bones of the foot. A subtle or mild variant may be present without an underlying condition (idiopathic) and occurs in about 10% to 20% of the population.[1] More commonly this malposition is the result of an underlying neuromuscular condition causing disruption of the normal balance of muscle tension holding the bones in place. The normal foot structure typically forms a tripod orientation between the first metatarsal head, calcaneus, and fifth metatarsal head, creating 3 points of contact. When this tripod is out of balance, there is tilting of 1 element of the tripod leading to an increased load on the other 2 points of contact and an increased arch of the foot.[2] Alteration of the tripod between the first and fifth metatarsal heads is often from neuromuscular dysfunction, such as a weakness in the tibialis anterior muscle, intrinsic foot muscles, and/or peroneus brevis muscle leading to imbalance and overpowering by the peroneus longus and posterior tibialis. The attachment of the peroneus longus at the metatarsals and medial cuneiform results in forefoot protonation and forced countercorrection into foot supination with ambulation.[3] Hammer toes, contracture of the plantar fascia and callous formation under the metatarsal heads can often be seen associated with pes cavus. The onset of symptoms may be noticeable at any age range and can vary depending on the mechanism or responsible neuromuscular condition. Investigation for an underlying etiology is warranted when this condition is severe, causes pain, or is causing dysfunction of gait. Neuromuscular diseases associated with pes cavus are the muscular dystrophies, hereditary ataxias (such as Friedreich ataxia), hereditary neuropathies (such as Charcot–Marie–Tooth disease), cerebral palsy, and other disorders or injury to the upper motor neuron unit in the spinal cord or brain. Investigation should be guided by clinical suspicion after obtaining a thorough examination with attention to coexistent signs and symptoms and gathering a comprehensive personal and family history, including age of onset and the time course of symptoms.

Pes planovalgus (or flat foot) is a deformity involving the foot that is caused by a flattening of the normal medial arch. Symptoms usually progress slowly over time, with overpronation of the foot owing to increased ligamentous laxity. The etiology is typically idiopathic or owing to mild muscular hypotonia, which is rarely from a neuromuscular disorder and is a common familial trait. During the physical examination, it is important for the examiner to determine if the arch is flexible or rigid. A flexible flat foot is more often physiologic or idiopathic, but can be pathologic when weakness, bony abnormalities, or other signs or symptoms are also present. A flexible flat foot has been further characterized into type I (functional flat foot), type II (hypermobile flat foot with associated ligamentous laxity and tight heel cords), and type III (flexible flat foot associated with tibialis posterior tendon dysfunction).[4] Type I, or functional flat foot, is usually not painful and develops slowly over time from forces causing heel eversion. Type II may be associated with other disorders of ligamentous laxity, such as Ehlers–Danlos syndrome, Marfan syndrome, trisomy 21, or osteogenesis imperfecta.[5,6] Pain can be present and the condition may arise from tarsal coalition, vertical talus, or an accessory navicular bone. Type III flat foot is associated with tibialis posterior tendon dysfunction and is uncommon before 20 years of age. It can be seen with overuse (such as in dancers, ice skaters, and runners) and typically patients complain of pain around the posteromedial ankle with swelling along the course of the tibialis posterior tendon. Partial tearing or avulsion is also possible as disease progresses if untreated. Rigid pes planus is present with decreased range of motion at the tarsal and subtalar joints and the arch does not increase with toe raising. The arch can become rigid with tarsal coalition, peroneal spasticity, or dysfunction of the tibialis posterior muscle and tendon. Diagnostic testing is typically reserved to plain radiographs or testing for connective tissue conditions if they are suspected.

## NERVE ENTRAPMENT AND COMPRESSION NEUROPATHIES
### Morton's Neuroma

Morton's neuroma is the term for entrapment of a common plantar digital nerve of the foot. The plantar digital nerve is the terminal branch of the tibial nerve. This entrapment neuropathy most commonly occurs between the third and fourth metatarsals, but may involve any intermetatarsal space.[7] The etiology of this condition is not understood fully, but may be due to nerve compression (tight shoes) or increased traction of the nerve owing to proximal collapse of the transverse arch. Typically, this condition causes painful ambulation that is worsened by wearing shoes, because they put compression on this area, further irritating the nerve. Patients usually complain of a burning pain that radiates to the toes. A common complaint is the sensation of a "rolled up sock" feeling under the forefoot when pressure is applied to the area. Mulder's sign occurs when pain is elicited with palpation between the affected metatarsal space. MRI or ultrasound examination of the foot can show an enlargement (inflammation) of the entrapped nerve if the lesion is moderate to severe in nature. Ultrasound tends to be the preferred modality as MRI has been shown to have a high false positive rate.[8]

### Baxter's (Inferior Calcaneal) Nerve Entrapment

The inferior calcaneal nerve (ie, Baxter's nerve) is typically the first branch off the lateral plantar nerve. This nerve travels between the abductor hallucis and quadratus plantae muscles in close proximity to the anterior aspect of the medial calcaneal tuberosity. Entrapment occurs when this nerve is compressed between these muscles or against the calcaneus (**Fig. 4**). This typically results in sharp radiating or shooting heel pain and numbness on the plantar aspect of the foot and heel, which is often attributed to plantar fasciitis. In Baxter's nerve entrapment, the tenderness is felt at the origin of the abductor hallucis muscle along the medial aspect of the foot whereas the pain of plantar fasciitis is often felt at the bottom of the heel where the plantar tendon inserts onto the calcaneus. Additionally, unlike plantar fasciitis, pain associated with entrapment tends to get worse with physical activity, rather than better. Further complicating the clinical picture, the inferior calcaneal nerve may occasionally become entrapped against the calcaneus owing to bone spurs (calcaneal enthesophytes). Risk factors for developing inferior calcaneal nerve entrapment include pes planus, obesity, older age, and having plantar fasciitis. Differentiation between inferior calcaneal nerve entrapment and plantar fasciitis is difficult and radiographs, ultrasound examination, and MRI can be used for aid in diagnosis, but only to rule out other possible conditions and risk factors. Local anesthetic injection to numb the inferior calcaneal nerve can result in effective relief of symptoms and is both diagnostic and therapeutic.[9]

### Tarsal Tunnel Syndrome

Tarsal tunnel syndrome arises from compression of the tibial nerve as it passes underneath the transverse tarsal ligament in the ankle. Along with this distal segment of the tibial nerve, the tendons of the flexor digitorum longus and flexor hallucis longus muscles, the vascular bundle, and the medial and lateral plantar nerves pass through this tunnel (**Fig. 5**). The most common cause of compression in this area arises from a fracture or dislocation involving the talus, calcaneus, or medial malleolus. Much less common etiologies of tibial nerve dysfunction include inflammation (such as seen with rheumatoid arthritis) and tumors. The typical presentation involves pain (aching or burning) and numbness or paresthesias of the sole of the forefoot (sometimes extends

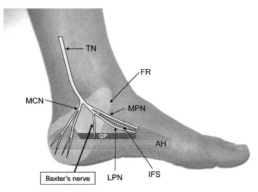

**Fig. 4.** Baxter's (inferior calcaneal) nerve entrapment. (*From* Del Toro D, Nelson PA. Guiding treatment for foot pain. Phys Med Rehabil Clin N Am 2018;29(4):783-92. doi: 10.1016/j.pmr.2018.06.012. Epub 2018 Sep 14. PMID: 30293631.)

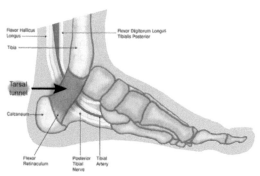

**Fig. 5.** Tarsal tunnel syndrome. (*From* Williams N, Willet J, Clark D, Ketteridge D. Tarsal tunnel syndrome in the mucopolysaccharidoses: A case series and literature review. JIMD Rep. 2019;46(1):16–22. Published 2019 Mar 14. https://doi.org/10.1002/jmd2.12021 https://onlinelibrary.wiley.com/doi/pdf/10.1002/jmd2.12021) CC BY 4.0.)

to the heel) and toes. Usually, these complaints are more prominent at night, worse after standing, and commonly there is pain with light sensory stimulation (allodynia) of the affected area making shoes or socks irritating to wear. Upon examination, a Tinel sign can be elicited over the tibial nerve posterior to the medial malleolus. Nerve conduction testing may reveal prolonged motor latencies in the tibial nerve with decreased conduction velocities across the flexor retinaculum.

### Fibular (Peroneal) Neuropathy

The fibular nerve, previously referred to as the peroneal nerve, is commonly injured as it crosses over the lateral aspect at the neck of the fibula (**Fig. 6**). External pressure may

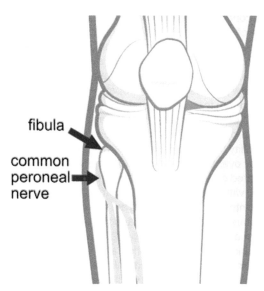

**Fig. 6.** Fibular nerve entrapment. (*From* https://www.kneeguru.co.uk/KNEEnotes/knee-dictionary/common-peroneal-nerve;Usedwithpermission.)

cause temporary dysfunction of the nerve, whereas chronic compression or trauma may cause demyelination, denervation, or transection of the nerve and would cause more long-lasting or even permanent deficits. The injury can come from a variety of causes including prolonged pressure to the nerve (such as with certain positioning during surgery or prolonged hospitalization), prolonged squatting or cross-legged sitting, tight leg casting, tight fitting clothing below the knee, blunt trauma, fibular fracture, or penetrating trauma. The symptoms of fibular nerve injury include foot drop causing a steppage gait. The patient frequently will have little to no ability to dorsiflex or evert the foot against gravity. Patients may also complain of paresthesias or numbness in the dorsum of the foot and lateral shin distal to the level of nerve injury. Pain is only reported in a minority of patients. Fibular nerve injury can also occur at the level of the ankle and rarely in the popliteal fossa. At the ankle, the compression is usually caused by a tight-fitting shoe or other strap around the ankle. In contrast with fibular nerve injury at the neck of the fibula, pain can be present with numbness most frequently described over the webspace between the first and second toes; weakness, if present, is minimal. Electromyography and nerve conduction studies can be useful for detecting conduction block of the fibular nerve past the site of injury. Distal motor and sensory response amplitudes can be decreased and may be absent in more severe cases with axonal injury. Abnormal muscle action potentials can be identified frequently in muscles innervated by the deep and superficial fibular nerves.[10]

## NEUROARTHROPATHY

Length-dependent sensory neuropathies often present with complaints of numbness in the feet selectively as the nerve endings are longer and further away from the neuron cell bodies. Loss of sensation may sometimes result in a chronic arthropathy leading to destruction and malformation of the foot joints that can cause substantial disability, pain, and difficulty with mobility. This disorder was coined by Dr Charcot when describing chronic arthritic changes to the feet of patients with tabes dorsalis and is aptly referred to as Charcot foot. Owing to the relative paucity of chronic syphilis in current culture, this condition is now most commonly seen in diabetes mellitus.

The pathogenesis of Charcot foot is often multifactorial, owing to several factors including mechanical, vascular, autonomic, and metabolic dysfunctions. Charcot foot classically presents after mild trauma with sudden onset of a unilateral warm, erythematous foot with edema over the foot and/or ankle. Other cases may be more insidious with slow progression of arthropathy over time. The typical morphology consists of a rocker bottom foot with collapse of the medial arch and medial displacement of the talonavicular joint or tarsometatarsal dislocation. (**Fig. 7**) Ligamentous laxity with a lack of proprioceptive stability is postulated to lead to increased joint movement and instability owing to a lack of inherent protective features. Repetitive minor (or micro) traumas over time, combined with impaired bone and joint repair mechanisms and exaggerated cytokine inflammatory response, can lead to a breakdown of the joint and bones, with destruction of the intrinsic foot architecture.[11] The most frequently involved joints in diabetic patients are the tarsus and tarsometatarsal joints, followed by the metatarsophalangeal joints and the ankle.[12] Bilateral and recurring attacks in the same foot are rare and only about 20% may have an attack in the contralateral foot. Pain is typically not severe during attacks (probably compounded by the sensory loss) and pain is poorly localized. Without treatment, progression can be rapid, and irreversible damage can occur within 6 months or less, resulting in severe and irreversible joint damage, further foot deformation, and alteration to weight bearing patterns that commonly cause additional skin ulcerations and infections.[13,14]

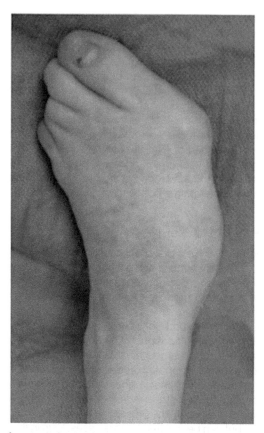

**Fig. 7.** The Charcot foot in diabetics. (*From* Frykberg RG, Zgonis T, Armstrong DG, et al. Diabetic foot disorders: A clinical practice guideline-2006 revision. The Journal of Foot and Ankle Surgery 2006;45(5):S1-S66.)

Overall, foot neuroarthropathy still tends to be a rare phenomenon, even in diabetic patients. There is an incidence of 0.3% per year in this patient group.[15] Chronic poorly controlled blood sugar levels tend to increase this likelihood. One study found that patients with type 1 diabetes presented more frequently in their fifth decade, with an average duration of disease of 24.0 ± 8.4 years, whereas type 2 diabetics tended to present in their sixth decade, with a mean duration of 13.0 ± 8.1 years.[16]

Although the stereotypical neuroarthropathy is considered to be Charcot foot, neuroarthropathy in other joints is also possible. Neuroarthropathy of the knees, hips, and ankles has been reported in patients with tabes dorsalis, and syringomyelia is classically associated with neuroarthropathy of the elbow. Other medical conditions that can cause neuroarthropathy include chemotherapy-induced neuropathy, vasculitic neuropathy, or any other longstanding idiopathic neuropathy.

The diagnosis of neuroarthropathy of the foot must be suspected early, because a delay in diagnosis can lead to disease progression and permanent disability without proper intervention. Any patient with a unilateral warm, swollen, and erythematous foot, especially if they have long-standing diabetes or other signs of sensory loss, should be evaluated for this disease process. It is important to differentiate Charcot foot from other conditions that present with similar symptoms. These conditions include septic arthritis, osteomyelitis, cellulitis, crystal-associated arthritis (gout or pseudogout), osteoarthritis, inflammatory arthritis, and complex regional pain syndrome. Radiographic findings of neuroarthropathy include mild signs of soft tissue swelling or osteopenia early in the course of disease. If plain radiographs are normal, then a noncontrast MRI should be obtained because waiting weeks for repeat plain radiography to show signs consistent with neuroarthropathy may delay diagnosis and treatment initiation. Bone scintigraphy, PET, or a computed tomography scan can also be used if MRI is not available or circumstances do not permit the use of this modality. As the neuroarthropathy progresses, there may be evidence of further bone breakdown with reduction of joint spaces, possible joint dislocation, and loss of the phalangeal and metatarsal heads on plain radiographs.[17] Laboratory testing and synovial fluid aspiration tends to be normal throughout the course of disease, but can be useful to help differentiate between Charcot foot and other disease states.

## IMMUNE-MEDIATED POLYNEUROPATHIES

Guillain–Barré syndrome (GBS) is a disorder caused by autoantibody-mediated demyelination and/or axon loss of peripheral nerves. Classically, the presentation starts with weakness and pain coming from dysfunction of the nerves distally (in the feet) and progressing proximally; however, there are several variants that may present with a different distribution of symptoms.

Acute inflammatory demyelinating polyneuropathy (AIDP) is the name of the most common form of GBS, whereas alterations in the underlying pathogenesis or distribution of symptoms have led to the named variants Miller–Fisher syndrome, polyneuritis cranialis, acute motor axonal neuropathy, and acute motor–sensory axonal neuropathy. GBS is usually an acute monophasic illness starting within a few days to weeks after an antecedent infection. Paresthesias in the feet followed by weakness and difficulty with ambulation is commonly the presenting complaint.[18] Signs and symptoms tend to be symmetric, but can be unilateral in rare cases. Pain in the legs and back and autonomic instability may also be present. The distribution and duration can be variable, with some patients only experiencing mild symptoms in the distal lower extremities, whereas others experience weakness that progresses rostrally to involve the hands and arms, trunk (causing breathing difficulty that may require mechanical ventilation), or face. The time to the peak of symptoms is typically less than 4 weeks and recovery is complete in most by 6 months; severe cases are reported to take 18 to 24 months to recover and severe disability without full recovery occurs in fewer than 5% of patients.[19,20] Chronic inflammatory demyelinating polyneuropathy (CIDP) is also a rare acquired autoimmune disorder of the peripheral nerves. It is distinguished from GBS by longer duration of illness (≥8 weeks for chronic inflammatory demyelinating polyneuropathy) and a relapsing/remitting nature. Classically, chronic inflammatory demyelinating polyneuropathy presents as an acute to subacute symmetric, motor > sensory neuropathy with weakness present in both proximal and distal muscles and with mild sensory loss and globally diminished or absent reflexes. CIDP can also have periodic relapses in a relapsing-remitting or relapsing-progressive pattern which typically doesn't happen in the monophasic illness of AIDP.

The initial diagnosis of GBS is based on the clinical presentation of progressive, symmetric ascending weakness with absent deep tendon reflexes. An analysis of the cerebrospinal fluid and electrodiagnostic studies is conducted in any patients with concern for GBS to ensure prompt diagnosis and treatment. On cerebrospinal fluid (CSF) analysis, an elevated CSF protein with a normal CSF white blood cell count is typically encountered. This finding, known as albuminocytologic dissociation, is present in more than 50% of patients within the first week and in more than 75% of patients by the third week. Nerve conduction studies and needle electromyography can be valuable for diagnostics and prognosis.[21] Demyelinating forms of GBS show decreased motor nerve conduction velocities, prolonged distal motor latency, increased F wave latencies, conduction block, and temporal dispersion.[22] Axonal forms of GBS have decreased distal motor and/or sensory amplitudes on nerve conduction studies. Enhancement and thickening of spinal nerve roots may be seen when a spinal MRI with gadolinium administration is performed. Serum IgG antibodies and CSF neuronal antibodies have been found in rare variants of GBS and, owing to the scarcity/lack of clinical usefulness, are not routinely tested for. A nerve biopsy can show peripheral nerve demyelination, but is not used very often anymore.

## HEREDITARY PERIPHERAL NEUROPATHIES

The hereditary peripheral neuropathies all present with a chronic progressive course of muscle weakness that is caused by mutations in genes involved in preserving the structure and function of Schwann cells, the myelinating cells of the peripheral nervous system. This heterogeneous group of disorders is classified based on clinical characteristics, mode of inheritance, electrophysiologic features, metabolic defects, and now more specifically with genetic markers.[23] The typical presentation of the hereditary peripheral neuropathies is slowly progressive distal weakness and atrophy of the intrinsic foot and calf muscles leading to foot drop, pes cavus, hammer toes, and a stork leg deformity (**Fig. 8**). Pain is not a predominant complaint, but sensory loss can often be present. The nomenclature was originally based on the prototypic hereditary neuropathy Charcot–Marie–Tooth disease; however, the clinical phenotypes, genetic defects, and underlying pathology can differ dramatically between different subtypes.[24] A brief review of the main clinical subtypes of these disorders is presented below followed by a summary on diagnostic evaluation and testing at the end of this section.

Classic Charcot–Marie–Tooth disease 1 is characterized by peripheral nerve demyelination and follows an autosomal-dominant pattern of inheritance. Patients typically

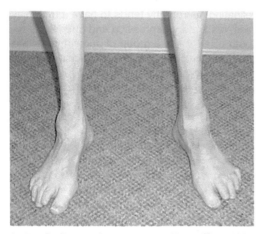

**Fig. 8.** Charcot–Marie–Tooth disease. (*From* Oster, DPM, Jeffrey. 2020. "CHARCOT MARIE TOOTH DISEASE." My Foot Shop. https://www.myfootshop.com/charcot-marie-tooth-disease#Tab3.)

present with symptoms that are slowly progressive and first noticed in the first or second decades. Decreased endurance with running (owing to weakness) and/or frequent sprained ankles may be reported. On examination, there may be areflexia, diminished sensory perception (vibration and proprioception), distal muscle weakness, pes cavus, and distal muscle atrophy with a tapering distribution (stork leg deformity). Late in the disease course, there can be hypertrophy of the peripheral nerves and palpable enlargement of the nerves can sometimes be appreciated on examination.

Charcot–Marie–Tooth disease 2 has a similar phenotype to Charcot–Marie–Tooth disease 1, with axonal damage characterized by distal weakness, atrophy, sensory loss, decreased deep tendon reflexes, and variable foot deformity. Sensory symptoms tend to be more prominent and palpable enlargement of peripheral nerves is not present. Onset is typically a little later than Charcot–Marie–Tooth disease 1, presenting in the second or third decade. Inheritance is typically autosomal dominant. An early onset, severe form of Charcot–Marie–Tooth disease 2 has been identified with onset in the first years of life, with rapidly progressive weakness and eventual full loss of the ability to ambulate.

Charcot–Marie–Tooth disease X subtypes are forms of hereditary neuropathy that affect primarily male patients. Carrier females are either mildly symptomatic or asymptomatic. Infantile to juvenile onset is typical with atrophy and weakness of lower leg muscles, areflexia, and pes cavus. Intellectual disability, dysphagia, dysarthria, and/or hearing loss have also been reported. Pain could be present in patients old enough to localize symptoms. These symptoms can occur as intermittent, stroke-like episodes that can be show reversible lesions on diffusion-weighted, T2, and fluid-attenuated inversion recovery sequences in the deep white matter, predominantly in the posterior brain regions or splenium of the corpus callosum on MRI.[23]

Charcot–Marie–Tooth disease 3 is confined to 2 particular clinical entities, Dejerine–Sottas syndrome and congenital hypomyelinating neuropathy. These disorders are characterized by a decreased production of normal myelin, resulting in thin, poorly formed or missing segments of myelination on peripheral nerves. Both disorders present in early infancy with pronounced hypotonia. There is typically more severe motor and sensory dysfunction with absent reflexes, hypotonia, and weakness that progresses proximally. Contractures can develop early or later as disease progresses. Congenital hypomyelinating neuropathy tends to have a more severe clinical course with feeding difficulties, respiratory depression and often leads to death in infancy.[25]

Charcot–Marie–Tooth disease 4 is a group of autosomal-recessive, demyelinating sensorimotor neuropathies. The clinical course is typically more severe than the autosomal dominant varieties (such as Charcot–Marie–Tooth disease 1). Distal muscle weakness is characteristic with atrophy and sensory loss leading to foot deformities and gait dysfunction.[26]

Hereditary neuropathy with liability to pressure palsy typically presents in the second decade, but may present anywhere between the first and third decades. Patients have symptoms of nerve dysfunction, such as weakness and/or paresthesias after compression of the nerve owing to minor trauma, which tends to resolve over the course of days to months. The most commonly affected nerves in this disorder are the peroneal, ulnar, radial, and axillary nerves along with the brachial plexus. Other findings may include cranial nerve involvement, sensorineural deafness, and scoliosis.

There are other small groupings of rare subtypes including hereditary motor and sensory neuropathy/Charcot–Marie–Tooth disease 5, 6, and 7, and an intermediate form of Charcot–Marie–Tooth disease with more being added with the discovery of new genetic markers and clinical phenotypes.[25]

A hereditary peripheral neuropathy should be suspected when the history and examination reveal slowly progressive weakness, gait abnormalities, decreased deep tendon reflexes, pes cavus, and/or hammer toes, as well as a diminished sensory perception on examination. The diagnostic evaluation of the hereditary peripheral neuropathies usually involves electrodiagnostics and genetic evaluation.[27] Electrodiagnostic testing typically involves 2 components, nerve conduction studies and needle electromyography. The nerve conduction study portion of the test shows signs of demyelination consisting of slowing of conduction velocities, prolonged distal latencies, prolonged F wave latencies, conduction block, and/or temporal dispersion in motor and sensory nerves. Needle electromyography examination is typically normal. If nerve conduction studies are normal, then Charcot–Marie–Tooth disease is not present and electromyographic findings may reveal the presence of a myopathy or disorder of the neuromuscular junction.[28]

Genetic testing has become a mainstay in the evaluation of the hereditary peripheral neuropathies. The unifying feature of these disorders is a mutation (deletion, duplication, or point mutation) in genes involved in the proper functioning of the myelin, axons and gap junctions of peripheral nerves. Autosomal dominant inheritance is characteristic of the classic forms (Charcot–Marie–Tooth disease 1A, 1B, 1C, etc), but as genetic testing has become more detailed and accessible, there has been expanding discovery of autosomal-recessive and X-linked forms. Peripheral myelin protein 22 (PMP22) on chromosome 17p11.2-p1 is the gene responsible for the classic form of Charcot–Marie–Tooth disease 1. Duplication or point mutations in this gene produce the phenotype of Charcot–Marie–Tooth disease, whereas deletions in this same gene lead to the phenotype of hereditary neuropathy with pressure palsy. Next-generation genetic sequencing panels dedicated to the hereditary peripheral neuropathies cover mutations in the 4 gene mutations responsible for more than 90% of hereditary neuropathy (PMP22, MPZ, GJB1, and MFN2) and all of the subtypes discussed in this article. The decreasing cost and widespread availability of this testing has led many clinicians to choose forgoing electrodiagnostic testing if there is a clear family history and the clinical picture is consistent with an hereditary peripheral neuropathy. Sporadic Charcot–Marie–Tooth disease caused by de novo mutations remains common, which makes the need for electrodiagnostic testing in many circumstances. Sural nerve biopsy is another testing modality that is used infrequently in current practice, but can show onion bulbing on histologic examination owing to repeated demyelination and remyelination over years.

## HEREDITARY ATAXIAS

The hereditary ataxias cause motor incoordination from cerebellar, spinal cord or ion channel dysfunction. These disorders are typically divided into 3 classes, progressive/degenerative ataxias, ataxias caused by disorders of metabolism, and episodic ataxias. Each group is characterized individually below.

### Progressive and Degenerative Ataxias

The progressive ataxias can follow an autosomal-dominant, autosomal-recessive, X-linked, or mitochondrial mode of inheritance.[29] Many of these come from a trinucleotide repeat expansion on the disease-causing gene rather than gene–protein mutations customary of most other hereditary neurologic conditions. The prototypical progressive ataxia is the autosomal dominant form of spinocerebellar ataxia. More than 40 spinocerebellar ataxias have been identified, classified by unique clinical and/or genetic abnormalities. The spinocerebellar ataxia variants with identifying clinical characteristics and associated gene loci are listed in **Table 1**. The most common trinucleotide repeat expansion is a CAG repeat that produces a toxic gain of function that exhibits an anticipatory expansion with each successive generation and leads to progressively earlier presentation and more severe symptoms.

Autosomal-recessive ataxias include Friedreich ataxia and ataxia-telangiectasia. Friedreich ataxia is caused by loss of function mutations in the frataxin gene (FXN) from GAA expansion repeats leading to reduced transcription and expression of the FXN gene.[30] Frataxin is a mitochondrial protein that is involved with iron homeostasis. In addition to the progressive ataxia and neurologic symptoms, patients may develop non-neurologic manifestations such as cardiomyopathy and diabetes mellitus. Symptoms typically present in the first decade, with a slowly progressive ataxic gait and distinct distal motor weakness. Loss of position and vibration sense is typically observed on physical examination and deep tendon reflexes are usually trace or absent. Bladder dysfunction may be reported along with other autonomic dysfunctions. Symptoms usually start in the feet and legs, but arm weakness, dysarthria, dysphagia, and truncal ataxia are typically seen as the disease progresses. Kyphoscoliosis is very common and can even precede neurologic symptoms. Pes cavus, equinovarus deformities, hammer toes, and atrophy of the intrinsic muscles of the feet is typically observed. Nerve conduction studies typically confirm an axonal sensory neuropathy with reduced or absent sensory nerve action potentials, and there may be mildly slowed motor conduction velocities. MRI of the neuraxis reveals atrophy of the spinal cord and medulla, as well as thinning of the dorsal nerve roots; however, cerebellar atrophy is uncommon. Diagnostic confirmation can be obtained through gene testing with either a next-generation gene sequencing panel or individual gene testing.

Ataxia-telangiectasia is a rare disorder that is characterized by progressive difficulty with coordinating movements (ataxia) beginning in early childhood, usually before age 5. Chorea, myoclonus, distal motor weakness, oculomotor apraxia, sensory deficits, and dysarthria are also typically seen. The movement problems generally progress causing wheelchair dependence by adolescence. Small clusters of enlarged blood vessels, called telangiectasias, occur in the eyes and on the surface of the skin and are also characteristic of this condition. People with ataxia-telangiectasia often have a weakened immune system, and many develop chronic lung infections. They also have an increased risk of developing cancer, particularly leukemia or lymphoma. Affected individuals tend to have high amounts of a protein called alpha-fetoprotein in their blood. The level of this protein is normally increased in the bloodstream of pregnant women, but it is unknown why individuals with ataxia-telangiectasia have elevated alpha-fetoprotein or what effects it has in these individuals. The life expectancy of people with ataxia-telangiectasia varies greatly, but affected individuals typically live into early adulthood. Ataxia-telangiectasia is caused by a mutation of the Ataxia Telangiectasia, Mutated (ATM) gene that is responsible for a protein kinase vital to inherent DNA damage repair.[31] The ATM protein is a large gene that can have different mutations causing a range of functional impacts to this DNA repair mechanism and correlates with the variable severity of disease in each individual. Xeroderma pigmentosum and Cockayne syndrome are less frequent causes of hereditary ataxia that also arise from defects in DNA repair mechanisms.

The X-linked progressive spinocerebellar ataxias are rare and some may have pure cerebellar symptoms, whereas others may have additional neurologic abnormalities present. The specific genetic alterations for these clinical subtypes has not been fully confirmed but follow an inheritance pattern consistent with X-linked dominant from family history. Although these X-linked diseases primarily are expressed in males, a small percentage of females have some symptoms because of skewed inactivation of the X chromosome bearing the normal allele. Aside from ataxia, clinical characteristics may include intellectual disability, visual loss, deafness, spasticity, sideroblastic anemia, and adrenal insufficiency.[32]

Mitochondrial disorders can present with ataxia that can be progressive or intermittent. Defects in mitochondrial metabolism from a variety of causes produce the symptoms in these disease states. The mitochondrial disorders with ataxia as a notable symptoms include Leigh syndrome, Kearns–Sayre syndrome, mitochondrial encephalopathy, lactic acidosis, and stroke-like episodes, neurogenic weakness with ataxia and retinitis pigmentosa, mitochondrial recessive ataxia syndrome, spinocerebellar ataxia with epilepsy, sensory ataxia neuropathy, dysarthria, ophthalmoplegia, myoclonic epilepsy myopathy sensory ataxia, and myoclonic epilepsy with ragged red fibers. Additional clinical characteristics can include developmental delay or psychomotor regression, external ophthalmoplegia, seizures, lactic acidosis, and hypotonia and/or weakness.

MRI may reveal bilateral lesions in the basal ganglia, thalamus, brainstem, or spinal cord. Peripheral neuropathy with decreased nerve conduction velocity and demyelination also are frequent findings.

### Ataxia from Inborn Errors of Metabolism

Many inborn errors of metabolism can present with ataxia as a symptom of a more broad clinical phenotype. The constellation of symptoms has classically been used to help direct the clinician to the particular metabolic defect and associated syndrome. For the sake of this review, these disorders can be divided into chronic progressive ataxias or intermittent ataxias and are listed in **Table 1**.

Symptom onset for these disorders ranges between infancy and adolescence. Intellectual disability, hypotonia, frequent illness, episodic vomiting, headaches, seizures, dermatitis, tremor, parkinsonism, eye movement abnormalities, and visual loss can also be seen along with the progressive ataxia. Biochemical screening usually is completed shortly after birth and is an effective way to test for many of these conditions. Metabolic testing may need to be collected later in life if the patient did not have this testing completed postnatally or if there is clinical suspicion of a false negative test on neonatal screening. Testing of individual genes or a gene panels is not frequently used as a first-line diagnostic testing owing to numerous mutations in a wide range of relevant genes making biochemical analysis more practical and cost efficient.

### Episodic Ataxias

Episodic ataxias represent a group of disorders that generally have onset in childhood or adolescence. The patients typically go through spells of ataxia that are provoked by physical exercise/exertion, stress, postural change, emotion, hunger, illness, or temperature change. Symptoms may also include myokymia (rippling of muscles), dysarthria, nystagmus, vertigo, nausea/vomiting, and tremor. Most affected individuals have normal or near normal neurologic function between attacks. These disorders arise from genetic defects causing dysfunction of ion channels, ion pumps, and glutamate transporters. Inheritance is sporadic or autosomal dominant. Researchers have identified at least 7 types of episodic ataxia, designated type 1 through type 7. The types are distinguished by their pattern of signs and symptoms, age of onset, length of attacks, and, when known, genetic cause. Mutations in the KCNA1, CACNA1A,

**Table 1**
**Hereditary ataxias due to errors of metabolism**

| Major Causes of Hereditary Ataxias Owing to Known Enzymatic Defects | |
|---|---|
| Disorder | Gene Locus and Protein |
| Intermittent ataxias | |
| Hyperammonemias and aminoacidurias | |
| Ornithine transcarbamylase deficiency | Xp21.1 | Ornithine transcarbamylase |
| Citrullinemia | 9q34 | Arginosuccinate synthetase |
| Arginase deficiency | 6q23 | Arginase |
| Argininosuccinic aciduria | 7cen-q11 | Arginosuccinate lyase |
| Hyperornithemia– hyperammonemia– homocitrullinuria syndrome | 13q14 | Mitochondrial ornithine transporter |
| Hartnup disease | 5p15.33 | Neutral amino acid transporter |
| Isovaleric acidemia | 15q14 | Isovaleric acid CoA dehydrogenase |
| Disorders of pyruvate and lactate metabolism | |
| Pyruvate dehydrogenase complex | Xp22.2 (most common) | E1-alpha subunit (most common) |
| Multiple carboxylase deficiency | 21q22 | Holocarboxylase synthetase |
| Progressive ataxias | |
| Tay–Sachs disease | 15q23-q24 | Alpha subunit of hexosaminidase A |
| Sandhoff disease | 15q13 | Beta subunit of hexosaminidase A and B |
| Niemann–Pick types A and B | 11p15.4-p15.1 | Acid sphingomyelinase |
| Niemann–Pick type C | 18q11-q12 14q24.3 | NPC1 NPC2 |
| Metachromatic leukodystrophy | 22q13 | Arylsulfatase A |
| Adrenomyeloneuropathy | Xq28 | Adrenoleukodystrophy protein |
| Abetalipoproteinemia | 4q22 | Microsomal triglyceride transfer protein |
| Hypobetalipoproteinemia | 2p24 | Apolipoprotein B |
| Cerebrotendinous xanthomatosis | 2q33 | Mitochondrial sterol 27-hydroxylase |
| Ataxia with vitamin E deficiency | 8q13 | Alpha-tocopherol transfer protein |
| Lesch–Nyhan syndrome | Xq26 | Hypoxanthine-guanine phosphoribosyl- transferase |
| Wilson disease | 13q14 | ATP7B (copper transporting ATPase) |
| Neuronal ceroid lipofuscinosis | Several variants | Multiple gene products |
| Refsum disease | 10pter | Phytanoyl CoA hydroxylase |
| X-linked ataxia, ichthyosis, and tapetoretinal dystrophy | Xpter-p22 | Arylsulfatase C |

CACNB4, and SLC1A3 genes have been associated with episodic ataxias 1, 2, 5, and 6, respectively.

## CEREBRAL PALSY (FOOT)

Cerebral palsy refers to a permanent but static impairment in motor function from a confirmed or presumed central nervous system insult. This impairment results in an impairment that primarily affects muscle tone, posture, and/or movement. The clinical presentation and etiology of cerebral palsy tends to be diverse. Insults to the developing nervous system may occur in utero (nuchal cord, maternal substance abuse, etc) and can happen during or shortly after the birthing process. Certain conditions put infants at an increased risk for cerebral palsy, including a history of prematurity, low birth weight, multiple gestation, in utero or perinatal infection, or known brain malformation. Although the underlying disorder does not progress or worsen, the clinical findings may change or worsen over time the central and peripheral nervous systems of the child matures and the musculature has abnormal signals for development. Clinical signs vary substantially and do not necessarily correlate with radiographic findings. Additional or associated findings in conjunction with the motor findings can be present, but are not present definitively. These finding include intellectual disability, altered sensory perception including auditory or visual disturbance, autonomic dysfunction, communication and language disabilities, neurobehavioral conditions, seizures, and/or musculoskeletal alterations.

The typical motor findings with cerebral palsy are increased muscle tone with impairment in voluntary movement evident by discoordination and/or restricted range of motion. This impairment may affect all limbs (quadriplegia), 1 side of the body (hemiplegia), upper limbs alone (paraplegia), or lower limbs alone (diplegia). Different movement abnormalities may be present instead of or in addition to these hypertonic-related movement abnormalities and include ataxia, choreoathetosis, or other dyskinesias (such as dysmetria or dystonia). Historically, a hypotonic variant of cerebral palsy was recognized previously, but has been excluded from more contemporary classifications. Muscular symptoms range from mild hypertonia to contracture. Muscle hypertonicity in cerebral palsy can vary, but more patterns would include degrees of elbow and knee flexion, adduction and internal rotation of the hips, and equinovalgus or calcaneovarus deformity in the foot. Atrophy of the musculature in the affected area is present frequently and correlates commonly with the degree of spasticity. Upper motor neuron signs are typically seen on physical examination and include hyper-reflexia, clonus, and/or persistence of extensor plantar response (Babinski reflex) and other primitive developmental reflexes. Developmental milestones are delayed frequently or never achieved, depending on disease severity. Delayed achievement of several developmental motor milestones are key markers for making the diagnosis and include not sitting by 8 months, not walking by 18 months, and early development of hand preference before 1 year of age. A diagnosis of cerebral palsy is typically confirmed between 12 and 24 months of age, but many physical signs may be present earlier in infancy. Subtle clinical characteristics or motor delays may occasionally lead to delayed diagnosis after 2 years of age.[33]

There is no particular diagnostic test that confirms the diagnosis of cerebral palsy and serial examinations are vital to making the correct diagnosis. However, several testing modalities can be helpful in aiding the clinician for diagnostic purposes. Brain imaging is typically the modality of choice for a diagnostic workup.

Although there is no specific timing to obtain this imaging, it is usually obtained earlier if the clinical history is recognized to be more severe or other diagnostic considerations warrant the testing. A brain MRI and head ultrasound examination have both been used for clinical imaging and provide their own benefits and detriments. Brain MRI can show signs of injury ranging from damage to the subcortical white matter (periventricular leukomalacia), cortical or intraventricular hemorrhage, or stroke. These findings on imaging do not always correlate well with clinical symptoms or prognostication owing to a wide range of possible outcomes. Shortly after birth, the brain has a much higher concentration of water content that prepares the brain for the birthing process, but causes decreased differentiation of discrete brain regions on MRI. As the infant grows, this water content decreases and the cortical structures and white matter tracts mature, leading to clearer visualization on imaging after 3 months with further improvement by 2 years of age. Imaging findings, along with the clinical history, can also be helpful in determining the need for additional diagnostic testing for alternate etiologies, including clotting disorders, infection, or inborn errors of metabolism. Cranial ultrasound examination is another useful neuroimaging modality that can show supratentorial structures to assess for hydrocephalus, cortical or ventricular hemorrhage, or brain malformation. Cranial ultrasound examination is a fast, noninvasive test that does not require any sedation; however, there is a limited view of the posterior head regions and requires that the infant still has open fontanelles. A brain MRI can initially be normal in patients later diagnosed with cerebral palsy and the timing and etiology of brain injury can not be determined in up to 90% of patients.[34] Additional testing may be warranted if there is not a clear etiology, neuroimaging is unrevealing, the clinical picture is not consistent with cerebral palsy, and/or there is clinical suspicion of possible alternate etiology. This workup can include laboratory testing consisting of a metabolic profile, thrombophilia evaluation, serum creatine kinase, ammonia, lactate, pyruvate, acylcarnitine profile, serum amino acids, and/or urine organic acids. Next-generation genetic sequencing has revealed a small but growing list of conditions that were previously thought to be idiopathic or cryptogenic. The diagnostic yield of genetic testing is increased if there are multiple organ systems also affected, dysmorphic features on examination or a family history of cerebral palsy. This testing can be particularly helpful for family planning or diagnostic closure for the family. Lumbar puncture is not routinely done for the workup of cerebral palsy, except in unusual cases where there is no clear etiology from history and all the abovementioned testing is reported as normal. Examination of the placenta for pathologic changes can also sometimes aid in the diagnostic workup of cerebral palsy.

## MUSCULAR DYSTROPHY

Neuromuscular disorders may also present with substantial weakness and/or lower extremity deformity. The presenting complaint is typically hypotonia, weakness, facial diplegia with feeding difficulties, respiratory dysfunction, and skeletal deformities such as arthrogryposis or club feet.[35] Associated symptoms may include cataracts, reduced vision or hearing, cognitive deficits, sleep disturbances, cardiac abnormalities, and endocrine disturbances. The onset of symptoms can be seen at birth for congenital muscular dystrophy and congenital myotonic dystrophy. Duchenne and Becker muscular dystrophies can present with weakness onset and difficulty ambulating around 2 years of age or after. Becker muscular dystrophy typically has a later onset and a milder phenotype. Laboratory testing usually reveals a very elevated creatine kinase level on serum testing. Brain imaging is typically normal, but some of the muscular dystrophies may have associated brain malformations, including Fukuyama type, Walker–Warburg syndrome, and muscle–eye–brain disease. These disorders all involve dysfunction of muscle function, which are caused by a genetic mutation that interferes with normal muscle function.[36,37] Duchenne and Becker muscular dystrophies arise from a mutation in the dystrophin gene on the X chromosome at Xp21. Myotonic dystrophy follows an autosomal-dominant inheritance pattern associated with mutation in the DMPK or CNBP genes and can follow an inticaperatory pattern across generations. Facioscapulohumeral muscular dystrophy is also autosomal dominantly inherited and arises from a defect in the DUX4 gene.

## DISCLOSURE

The authors has no commercial interest or financial support to disclose.

## REFERENCES

1. Seaman T. Pes cavus. Treasure. Island, FL: StatPearls Publishing; 2021. p. 32310476.
2. Wapner KL. Foot and ankle disorders: pes cavus. Philadelphia, PA: WB Saunders; 2000. p. 919–41.
3. Krähenbühl N. Anatomy and biomechanics of cavovarus deformity. Foot Ankle Clin 2019;24:173–81. https://doi.org/10.1016/j.fcl.2019.02.001.
4. Raj MA. Pes planus. Treasure Island, FL: StatPearls Publishing; 2021. p. NBK430802.
5. Techdijan MO. Clinical pediatric orthopedics: the art of diagnosis and the principles of management. Philadelphia: Appleton and Lange; 1997.
6. Toye MD, Leon R. "Baxter's nerve (first branch of the lateral plantar nerve) impingement." MRI Web Clinic 2012 (August): 1. 2012. Available at: https://radsource.us/baxters-nerve/.
7. Locke RK. Morton's neuroma. J Am Podiatr Med Assoc 1993;2:108–9. https://doi.org/10.7547/87507315-83-2-108.
8. Fazal MA. Ultrasonography and magnetic resonance imaging in the diagnosis of Morton's neuroma. J Am Podiatr Med Assoc 2012;102:184–6. https://doi.org/10.7547/1020184.
9. Presley JC. Sonographic visualization of the first branch of the lateral plantar nerve (Baxter nerve): technique and validation using perineural injections in a cadaveric model. J Ultrasound Med 2013;32(9):1643.
10. Poage C. Peroneal nerve palsy: evaluation and management. J Am Acad Orthop Surg 2016;24(1):1–10.
11. Petrova NL. Inflammatory and bone turnover markers in a cross-sectional and prospective study of acute Charcot osteoarthropathy. Diabet Med 2015;32: 267–73. https://doi.org/10.1111/dme.12590.
12. Dardari D. An overview of Charcot's neuroarthropathy. J Clin Transl Endocrinol 2020;22. https://doi.org/10.1016/j.jcte.2020.100239.
13. Rajbhandari SM. Charcot neuroarthropathy in diabetes mellitus. Diabetologia . 2002;45:1085–96. https://doi.org/10.1007/s00125-002-0885-7.
14. Rogers LC. The Charcot foot in diabetes. Diabetes Care 2011;9:2123–9. https://doi.org/10.2337/dc11-0844.

15. Petrova NL. Difference in presentation of Charcot osteoarthropathy in type 1 compared with type 2 diabetes. Diabetes Care 2004;27:1235–6. https://doi.org/10.2337/diacare.27.5.1235-a.

16. Fabrin J. Long-term follow-up in diabetic Charcot feet with spontaneous onset. Diabetes Care 2000;23:796–800. https://doi.org/10.2337/diacare.23.6.796.

17. Wukich DK. Charcot arthropathy of the foot and ankle: modern concepts and management review. J Diabetes Complications 2009;23:409–26. https://doi.org/10.1016/j.jdiacomp.2008.09.004.

18. Yuki N. Guillain-Barré syndrome. N Engl J Med 2012;24(366):2294–304.

19. Souayah N. National Trends in hospital Outcomes Among patients with Guillain-Barre syndrome requiring mechanical ventilation. J Clin Neuromuscul Dis 2008; 1(10):24–8. https://doi.org/10.1097/CND.0b013e3181850691.

20. Studler U. Fibrosis and adventitious bursae in plantar fat pad of forefoot: MR imaging findings in asymptomatic volunteers and MR imaging-histologic comparison. Radiology 2008;3(246):863. https://doi.org/10.1148/radiol.2463070196.

21. Hadden RD. Electrophysiological classification of Guillain-Barré syndrome: clinical associations and outcome. Plasma exchange/sandoglobulin Guillain-Barré syndrome trial group. Ann Neurol 1998;5:780–8. https://doi.org/10.1002/ana.410440512.

22. Uncini A. Electrodiagnostic criteria for Guillain-Barrè syndrome: a critical revision and the need for an update. Clin Neurophysiol 2012;123:1487–95. https://doi.org/10.1016/j.clinph.2012.01.025.

23. Pareyson D. New developments in Charcot-Marie-Tooth neuropathy and related diseases. Curr Opin Neurol 2017;30:471–80. https://doi.org/10.1097/WCO.0000000000000474.

24. Klein CJ. Inherited neuropathies: clinical overview and update. Muscle Nerve 2013;48:604–22. https://doi.org/10.1002/mus.23775.

25. Bird TD. Charcot-Marie-Tooth neuropathy type 4." gene reviews. Available at: https://www.ncbi.nlm.nih.gov/books/NBK1468/.

26. Bansagi B. Genetic heterogeneity of motor neuropathies. Neurology 2017;88: 1226–34. https://doi.org/10.1212/WNL.0000000000003772.

27. Saporta MA. Charcot-Marie-Tooth disease and other inherited neuropathies. Continuum 2014;20:1208–25. https://doi.org/10.1212/01. CON.0000455885.37169.4c.

28. Roy EP. Longitudinal conduction studies in hereditary motor and sensory neuropathy type 1. Muscle Nerve 1989;12:52–5. https://doi.org/10.1002/mus.880120110.

29. Brusse E. Diagnosis and management of early- and late-onset cerebellar ataxia. Clin Genet 2007;71:12–24. https://doi.org/10.1111/j.1399-0004.2006.00722.x.

30. Synofzik M. Autosomal recessive cerebellar ataxias: paving the way toward targeted molecular Therapies. Neuron 2019;101:560–83. https://doi.org/10.1016/j.neuron.2019.01.049.

31. Fogel BL. Clinical features and molecular genetics of autosomal recessive cerebellar ataxias. Lancet Neurol 2007;6:245–57. https://doi.org/10.1016/S1474-4422(07)70054-6.

32. Hagerman R. Advances in clinical and molecular understanding of the FMR1 premutation and fragile X-associated tremor/ataxia syndrome. Lancet Neurol 2013; 12:786–98. https://doi.org/10.1016/S1474-4422(13)70125-X.

33. Novak I. Early, accurate diagnosis and early intervention in cerebral palsy: advances in diagnosis and treatment. JAMA Pediatr 2017;171:897–907. https://doi.org/10.1001/jamapediatrics.2017.1689.

34. Krägeloh-Mann I. The role of magnetic resonance imaging in elucidating the pathogenesis of cerebral palsy: a systematic review. Dev Med Child Neurol 2007;49(2):144–51. https://doi.org/10.1111/j.1469-8749.2007.00144.x.
35. Griggs RC. Evaluation and treatment of myopathies. Philadelphia: Davos; 1995.
36. Hedge M. Microarray-based mutation detection in the dystrophin gene. Hum Mutat 2008;29:1091–9. https://doi.org/10.1002/humu.20831.
37. Turan I. Tarsal tunnel syndrome. Outcome of surgery in longstanding cases. Clin Orthop Relat Res 1997;343:151–6.

# Surgical Management of Foot and Ankle Deformities in Cerebral Palsy

Tamir Bloom, MD[a],*, Sanjeev Sabharwal, MD, MPH[b,c]

## KEYWORDS

- Cerebral palsy • Planovalgus • Equinovarus • Equinus • Foot deformities

## KEY POINTS

- Foot and ankle deformities in children with cerebral palsy develop over time because of dynamic muscle imbalance and abnormal biomechanics.
- As deformities progress, they may cause pain as well as compromise standing, ambulation, skin integrity, and brace tolerance.
- The goal of surgical management is to optimize foot shape and improve shock absorption function by correcting intrasegmental and intersegmental malalignment.
- It is important to address all pathologic segmental malalignments at the time of surgery by realigning the joints with soft-tissue releases, correcting bony deformities, and finally appropriate muscle balancing.
- When necessary, muscle fascia and intramuscular lengthening are favored over muscle releases and tendon lengthening, and osteotomy is preferred over arthrodesis to restore foot skeletal segmental alignment.

## INTRODUCTION

Cerebral palsy (CP) is the most common cause of physical disability in childhood, with a prevalence of approximately 1 in 500 neonates in most developed countries and an estimated worldwide prevalence of 17 million people.[1] CP is not a single entity but a group of diverse disorders with variable severity that stem from a lesion to the motor systems, and many times other regions, of the developing brain. The key features of CP include the following: (1) the lesion to the immature brain (within the first 3 years of life) is nonprogressive and permanent; (2) the lesion causes a disorder of movement and posture that limits activity; (3) the lesion affects musculoskeletal development throughout childhood leading to secondary and frequently progressive

[a] The Pediatric Orthopedic Center, 218 Ridgedale Avenue, Cedar Knolls, NJ 07927, USA; [b] UCSF Pediatric Orthopaedic Fellowship, University of California, San Francisco, 1500 Owens Street, San Francisco, CA 94158, USA; [c] Limb Lengthening and Reconstruction Center, UCSF Benioff Children's Hospital, 744 52nd Street, Oakland, CA 94609, USA
* Corresponding author.
E-mail address: tamirbloommd@gmail.com

Clin Podiatr Med Surg 39 (2022) 37–55
https://doi.org/10.1016/j.cpm.2021.09.001
podiatric.theclinics.com

musculoskeletal deformities; and (4) accompanying disturbances in sensation, perception, cognition, communication, and behavior.[2,3]

Children with CP are at a high risk of developing foot and ankle deformities that can impact function and seating.[4] The various neuromusculoskeletal pathologies in CP include impaired balance, poor coordination, sensory deficits, weakness, hypertonia, growth inhibition of muscle-tendon units and long bones, and progressive muscle abnormalities related to neuronal, nutritional, and mechanical factors.[5] This complex array of factors results in a spectrum of phenotypically variable foot and ankle abnormalities that can alter gait biomechanics and reduce functional activity. This article reviews some of the common foot and ankle deformities that occur in children with CP. Over the past 20 years, there have been important developments in the understanding and care of these problems, as well as continued evolution of new paradigms for clinical decision-making regarding surgery. Preferred operative procedures based on a review of the literature will be discussed. Surgical techniques and postoperative protocols are beyond the scope of this discussion.

Paramount to planning orthopedic care for children with CP is understanding their motor function and predicting their future motor function. The Gross Motor Functional Classification System (GMFCS) is useful for this purpose. The GMFCS is a reliable, valid, and practical method that divides the continuum of functional mobility in children and young adults with CP into 5 discrete groups (**Fig. 1**).[6,7] The GMFCS describes the child's functional abilities and their need for assistive mobility devices. Children with GMFCS level I have minimal functional limitations. They can run and jump but have mild impairments with balance, speed, and coordination. Children with GMFCS level II have limited ability to run and jump and have problems ascending and descending stairs. Children with GMFCS level III are usually using ankle foot orthosis (AFO) and crutches or walkers to ambulate, and often use manual powered wheelchairs for long distances. Children with GMFCS level IV usually require physical assistance or powered mobility in most settings but may be able to stand for short periods with assistance. They may walk short distances at home with physical assistance or a body-type walker. Children with GMFCS level V have severe physical impairment, require total care, and are dependent on others for mobility.

The GMFCS describes the prognosis, with most children improving in their gross motor function until they are about 6 years old.[8] Therefore, any intervention done at this time will appear to improve their function when in fact the improvements are predicted as corresponding to the natural history. In GMFCS levels III to V, there is a tendency for the GMFCS to decline coinciding with the onset of the adolescent growth.[9] Beginning at about 8 or 9 years of age, progressive foot and ankle deformities are common in diplegic and quadriplegic patients and may partially accounts for the deterioration of gait and GMFCS level.[10]

The GMFCS helps predict the development and progression of many of the musculoskeletal issues in CP (eg, contractures, decreased mobility, hip instability, deformities of the spine) and understand the outlook for a child's gross motor function with respect to children of similar age and severity. In addition, the GMFCS helps in educating families, therapists, and other health care professionals as to the extent surgical interventions improve function with respect to child's age and classification level. Although the GMFCS is not an outcome measure, the goal of lower extremity musculoskeletal surgery is to improve or at least maintain the child at the GMFCS level, and thus optimizing their overall level of function.[11]

Orthopedic surgery is a common component in the management of foot and ankle deformities in children with CP. However, surgery is rarely needed in the first few years of life (birth to age 4–6 years).[12] This early stage is characterized by abnormal movement

# GMFCS E & R between 6th and 12th birthday: Descriptors and illustrations

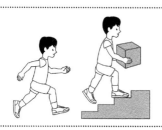

## GMFCS Level I

Children walk at home, school, outdoors and in the community. They can climb stairs without the use of a railing. Children perform gross motor skills such as running and jumping, but speed, balance and coordination are limited.

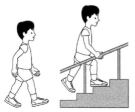

## GMFCS Level II

Children walk in most settings and climb stairs holding onto a railing. They may experience difficulty walking long distances and balancing on uneven terrain, inclines, in crowded areas or confined spaces. Children may walk with physical assistance, a hand-held mobility device or used wheeled mobility over long distances. Children have only minimal ability to perform gross motor skills such as running and jumping.

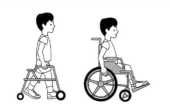

## GMFCS Level III

Children walk using a hand-held mobility device in most indoor settings. They may climb stairs holding onto a railing with supervision or assistance. Children use wheeled mobility when traveling long distances and may self-propel for shorter distances.

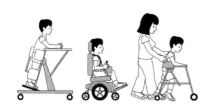

## GMFCS Level IV

Children use methods of mobility that require physical assistance or powered mobility in most settings. They may walk for short distances at home with physical assistance or use powered mobility or a body support walker when positioned. At school, outdoors and in the community children are transported in a manual wheelchair or use powered mobility.

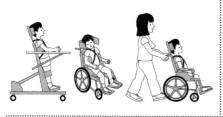

## GMFCS Level V

Children are transported in a manual wheelchair in all settings. Children are limited in their ability to maintain antigravity head and trunk postures and control leg and arm movements.

GMFCS descriptors: Palisano et al. (1997) Dev Med Child Neurol 39:214-23    Illustrations Version 2 © Bill Reid, Kate Willoughby, Adrienne Harvey and Kerr Graham,
CanChild: www.canchild.ca    The Royal Children's Hospital Melbourne   ERC151050

**Fig. 1.** The GMFCS as depicted for children age 6 to 12 years. (*From* Palisano et al. Dev Med Child Neurol 1997;39:214-23. CanChild: www.canchild.ca. Illustrations copyright @ Kerr Graham, Bill Reid and Adrienne Harvey, The Royal Children's Hospital, Melbourne.)

patterns (most commonly spasticity), few contractures, and delays in the acquisition of gross motor function. Young children usually have mild and flexible deformities with a variable and unpredictable natural history. Management primarily includes a combination of physical therapy, orthotic support, assistive devices, and spasticity management (oral medications, botulinum toxin A injections for focal spasticity, eg, spastic equinus). Neurosurgical management of spasticity with selective dorsal rhizotomy and intrathecal baclofen pump placement may be indicated at this time. Gait maturation usually occurs by 7 years of age.[13] Thus, surgical treatment for the foot and ankle in young children leads to limited improvement over the natural history of functional ability. Furthermore, orthopedic surgery at this age may cause unpredictable results, increased risk of recurrence, and lead to potentially adverse outcomes.[14–17]

After age 6 to 8 years, deformities of the foot and ankle are prone to progress because of persistent dynamic muscle imbalance and/or overactivity, impaired selective motor control, the development of soft-tissue contractures, and the progressive mismatch between the length of muscle-tendon units with respect to the adjacent long bone segment. With continued growth into adolescence, dynamic deformities become rigid involving a mixture of soft-tissue contractures, joint segmental malalignment, and osseous deformities. Worsening deformity and loss of foot flexibility can result in pain, skin irritation, poor brace tolerance, and gait deterioration. A multitude of deformities are observed, including a continuum from varus to valgus hindfoot malalignment. The kinematic coupled motion of the subtalar joint leads to 3 commonly observed foot and ankle segmental malalignment patterns: equinus, equinoplanovalgus, and equinocavovarus. Equinovarus usually occurs with some degree of forefoot adduction and pronation; equinovalgus with forefoot abduction and supination. Secondary deformities, such as ankle valgus and hallux valgus, may accompany pes valgus; toe flexion deformities may accompany severe equinus deformity. Each of these deformities disrupts normal foot function in a unique way,[18] and they will be discussed individually. Surgical management is often necessary to address progressive deformities.

In ambulatory children with CP (GMFCS I to III), the goal of surgical treatment is to achieve a plantigrade, braceable foot while maximizing mobility for shock absorption during loading response in the stance phase and maximally preserving muscle power. The surgical strategy includes correcting segmental malalignment, muscle imbalance, and biomechanical lever arm dysfunction. It is presumed that by achieving these goals, the function of the foot will be optimized by optimizing the prerequisites of normal gait, such as stability in stance, swing phase clearance, preposition of the foot in terminal swing, and energy conservation. In nonambulatory children, the goal of treatment is to maintain adequate foot shape to allow comfortable shoe wear and brace fit, potentially allowing therapeutic standing, and positioning in a wheelchair. Timely surgical intervention may reduce the risk of deformity progression, eliminate pain, and decrease the possibility of early degenerative arthrosis in adulthood. The challenges of surgical management of foot deformities in children with CP include the following: (1) determining appropriate surgical interventions; (2) optimal timing of surgery; (3) setting realistic goals of the patient, caregivers, and therapists; (4) coordinating care among a multidisciplinary team of health care providers; and (5) combining correction of the foot and ankle with other indicated lower extremity procedures under the same surgical encounter (single-event multilevel surgery [SEMLS]).

## EVALUATION AND CLINICAL DECISION-MAKING FOR SURGERY

Assessment of foot deformities in CP is multifaceted, requiring the collection and integration of data from a combination of sources that include the clinical history, standardized physical examination, observational and quantitative gait analysis, GMFCS classification, and radiographic findings.[19] If operative management is indicated, examination under anesthesia may also provide valuable information regarding the extent of dynamic deformity versus myostatic soft-tissue contractures. Information gleaned from each of these sources helps in understanding the natural history of the deformity, amount of soft-tissue imbalance and skeletal deformity, impact on gait dysfunction, and ultimately determining the optimal surgical treatment for that patient.

### Clinical History and Physical Examination

Children with foot deformities and their caregivers may report decreased walking ability, in-toeing or out-toeing, pain with ambulation, difficulty with shoe wear or orthoses fit, and deformity progression. A thorough "orthopedic" neurologic examination should be performed to describe and classify abnormalities in muscle strength and tone, abnormal movement patterns, the geographic pattern of involvement, and gross motor function.

The primary motor deficit is important to consider as it helps to understand the natural history as well as the outcome of surgical treatment. The most common movement disorder in CP is hypertonia (increased muscle tone), of which spasticity is the dominant pattern (77%–93%).[20] Spasticity is defined as a velocity-dependent increased resistance to passive muscle stretch. The second largest group of movement disorders in CP are dyskinesias (2%–15%). Dyskinesia is characterized by involuntary movements of the limbs and may coexist with spasticity (mixed type). Dyskinetic CP is associated with damage to the basal ganglia and thalamus and includes dystonia and less commonly choreoathetosis.[21] Dystonia is defined as a "movement disorder in which involuntary sustained or intermittent muscle contractions cause twisting and repetitive movements, abnormal postures, or both."[22] Compared to children with spastic CP, surgical outcomes of foot and ankle deformities in children with dyskinesias and mixed type commonly are more unpredictable.[1,23] In general, complete or partial tendon transfers are generally avoided in children with dystonia or mixed tone.[24] Children with ataxia and hypotonia (4% to 10%) often have cerebellar dysfunction and difficulties with balance and coordination. They rarely developed fixed contractures and surgical management is uncommon.

The geographic (or topographic, part of the body involved) classification includes either diplegia, hemiplegia, double hemiplegia, or quadriplegia. The intraobserver and interobserver error in the use of this classification scheme is high, and children younger than 5 or 6 years may be difficult to accurately classify. However, this classification is important to help identify involved limb segments and in understanding the natural history of the foot deformity. For example, the natural history of equinovarus deformity in children with hemiplegia is for the deformity to persist, whereas in a child with diplegia, equinovarus deformity tends to overcorrect into valgus.[25] Planovalgus feet are the most common foot deformity in children with spastic diplegia and quadriplegia.

Physical examination includes methodical evaluation of the hips, knees, and ankles with the child barefoot and wearing shorts. Evaluation of the foot and ankle should document the relationship among the forefoot, midfoot, and hindfoot in both weight-bearing and non–weight-bearing conditions. Range of motion and individual muscle strength and selective control of the involved limb segments are assessed. Equinus deformity to assess contractures of the gastrocnemius and/or soleus should be assessed with the foot inverted to lock the subtalar joint. The foot should be inspected for the presence of excessive or inadequate skin callus, which indicates disrupted loading patterns or problems with shoe or orthotic wear. Standing lower limb alignment (in the ambulatory patient) and rotational profile of the lower extremity should be assessed as this may affect foot posture.

Observational gait analysis is assessed, including the entire lower extremities in the sagittal, coronal, and transverse plane. Gait should be observed in multiple planes by having the child walked toward, away from, and past the examiner. Foot progression angle with respect to the pelvic rotation should be noted. Key events of the gait cycle that may be appreciated include foot position at initial contact (heel strike, flat foot, or toe strike), foot alignment in midstance (varus, neutral, or valgus) and swing-phase foot clearance should be noted.[18]

### Imaging and Advanced Modalities

Three (simulated) weight-bearing radiographs views of the foot and an AP view of the ankle should be obtained. Davids and colleagues described a comprehensive radiographic analysis using 10 radiographic measurements in the normal pediatric foot to aid in understanding segmental malalignment.[26] Individual measurements of segmental alignment can then be compared to normative values and ranges (values beyond 1 standard deviation from the normal mean value considered abnormal), and malalignment patterns can be described.

Instrumented 3-dimensional gait analysis (3DGA) provides a comprehensive evaluation of gait that includes joint kinematics (joint motions: position, angle, velocity, and acceleration of body segments and joint), joint kinetics (joint forces-ground reaction forces that moment), and electromyography (EMG). 3DGA when combined with a standard physical examination, that includes muscle strength and tone assessment, yields a "more complete picture" of gait abnormalities than when the static physical examination is used in isolation.[27] 3DGA is routinely used in ambulatory children with CP to assess gait pathology, and when multilevel surgery and/or rotational osteotomies are being considered. The complex anatomy and biomechanics of the foot make data derived from gait analysis of limited use for clinical decision-making for children with CP, if used in isolation. In a subset of patients with equinovarus deformity, dynamic EMG is particularly useful in determining the relative contribution of the tibialis anterior (TA) and tibialis posterior (TP) muscle forces during the gait cycle. This information facilitates clinical decision-making as to which muscle-tendon unit should be selected for lengthening or transfer.[28,29] Dynamic pedobarography can also be used in characterizing abnormal foot loading patterns and deformity severity of varus and valgus foot deformities.[30]

## SURGICAL PRINCIPLES

Treatment should be tailored to each individual child. Surgical procedures are determined by identifying all segmental malalignments and assessing the contribution of dynamic or flexible soft-tissue imbalance, fixed soft-tissue imbalance, and skeletal deformities. The initial surgical step is to realign all joint malalignments with a combination of capsular releases and/or plication, and musculotendinous unit lengthening. Skeletal deformities can be corrected with osteotomies or arthrodesis. Bony surgery can improve alignment by lengthening, shortening, angulation, or rotation. Whenever possible, osteotomy is preferred to arthrodesis to preserve foot joint mobility, shock absorption, function, and decrease the risk of adjacent segment arthrosis.[31] Muscle imbalance can be addressed with partial (split) or complete tendon transfers. Tendon transfers and capsular plication should be performed following the correction of bony deformities in a single surgical setting.

Surgical correction of foot and ankle deformities should be performed in conjunction with procedures to correct coexisting deformities of the lower extremities in one surgical setting. SEMLS is a concept that dates back to the 1980s and has become the gold standard for surgical treatment in children with CP.[32,33] The advantages of SEMLS include a single hospital admission, decreased need for repeated anesthetics, a single stay in inpatient rehabilitation, and the prevention of secondary deformities from delay in sequential treatment of spasticity, contractures, and bone deformities.[34] SEMLS is indicated in older children who have demonstrated functional decline or gait deviations warranting intervention.[35] Nonoperative treatment modalities (eg, spasticity management, orthoses, casting, physical therapy) should also be incorporated as part of SEMLS treatment, rather than sequentially, to optimize gait. Immobilization following surgical procedures, when required, should be limited to facilitate rehabilitation. For optimal outcomes, it is essential to set realistic goals for patients, caregivers, and therapists via a multidisciplinary team approach. Preparing the patient and family for surgery should also include discussions of postoperative rehabilitation, postoperative pain management, general anesthesia, medical costs, postoperative immobilization, and orthosis wear.

## EQUINUS DEFORMITY

Pure plantar flexion malalignment or equinus is the most common foot and ankle deformity seen in patients with CP. Selecting the appropriate surgical procedure requires understanding of the degree of fixed versus dynamic contracture and the relative contributions of the gastrocnemius (GSC) versus soleus via the Silverskold test.[36] Any associated forefoot plantar flexion deformity (cavus) should be identified on clinical examination and standing lateral radiographs of the foot. Surgical correction is indicated for equinus contractures that cannot be dorsiflexed past neutral, are refractory to nonoperative measures, and cause gait disturbance or brace intolerance.

Any attempt at surgical correction of equinus deformity risks the possibility of overcorrection (calcaneus), undercorrection, and recurrent equinus. Determining the amount of lengthening required and risks of surgery highlights the principle of "surgical dosing," which is a critical factor in selecting the appropriate procedure. Commonly used plantar flexion muscle group lengthening procedures can be grouped based on anatomic zones and their associated "dosage effect" (**Table 1**).[37] Proximal procedures that do not involve release of the soleus muscle fibers preserve the most push-off power but produce the least lengthening. They are associated with a low risk of overcorrection and an increased risk of recurrence.[38,39] Achilles tendon lengthening procedures can produce almost an unlimited amount of lengthening but a greater degree of weakness and surgical overcorrection.[40] Recurrent equinus can be readily surgically corrected. However, overlengthening of the Achilles tendon often leads to disabling calcaneus deformity with no predictable treatment. It is therefore recommended to err on the side of slight undercorrection when performing surgery for equinus contracture in such children, with the goal of achieving 5° of ankle dorsiflexion with the knee is extended.

In addition to the location of lengthening procedure, the risk of surgery also varies according to the motor type of CP, deformity severity, the age of the patient at index surgery, and the length of patient follow-up.[17,41] In general, surgical lengthening of the plantar flexion muscle groups in children older than 6 to 8 years have more predictable outcomes, with a lower risk of recurrent equinus than those operated under the age of

**Table 1**
Common surgical procedures for equinus deformity

| Anatomic Zone of the GSC Unit | Surgical Procedure Eponym | Description | Indications | Advantages & Disadvantages |
|---|---|---|---|---|
| Zone 1: GSC muscle belly | Baumann | Proximal GSC fascia recession Distal GSC fascia recession | • Only GSC involved, <20° of equinus with the knee extended that improves by >15° with the knee flexed | • Preserves muscle power and low risk of overcorrection<br>• Stable, last for immediate weight-bearing and cast |
| Zone 2: GSC and soleus musculotendinous junction | Modified Vulpius | Combined GSC and soleus (conjoined tendon) aponeurosis lengthening | • Both GSC and soleus involved with 20° or more correction required when EUA at the time of surgery<br>• Usually, spastic hemiplegia | • Stable, allows for immediate weight-bearing in cast |
| | Strayer | Isolated GSC aponeurosis lengthening | • Only GSC involved and up to 20° of equinus with the knee extended that improves by >15° with the knee flexed<br>• Usually, spastic diplegia | • Stable, allows for immediate weight-bearing in cast |
| | Gage modification of Strayer | Combined GSC and soleus aponeurosis lengthening | • Residual equinus deformity present following Strayer procedure | • Stable, allows for immediate weight-bearing in cast |
| Zone 3: Achilles tendon | | Achilles tendon lengthening | • Both GSC and soleus involved with >30° correction required | • May result in loss of muscle power and greater risk of overcorrection. Open tendon lengthenings may require non–weight-bearing and longer rehabilitation |

*Abbreviations:* EUA, examination under anesthesia; GSC, gastrocnemius muscle.

6 years. In young children with spastic diplegia, equinus results from overactivity of the gastrosoleus muscle in relation to the ground reaction force, rather than a weak TA.[41] The natural history in these children as they get older is a tendency to develop a crouch gait as the ground reaction force to overcome the moment arm generated by the gastrosoleus muscle.[42] In addition, children with spastic CP with equinus gait have longer than normal Achilles tendons and shorter than normal muscle bellies.[43] Therefore, when surgical correction of equinus gait is indicated in children with spastic diplegics, either GSC facia recession or GSC aponeurotic (+/− soleus fascia) lengthening are generally preferred over more extensive muscle releases and distal tendon lengthening.[44] These soft-tissue procedures minimize the risk of over-lengthening and weakening the posterior compartment musculature and result in more predictable improvement in ankle function. Ill-advised isolated tendon lengthenings in these patients may result in (pseudo)crouch gait with excessive ankle dorsiflexion in the stance phase causing gait dysfunction.[36,45]

In patients with spastic hemiplegia, equinus deformity often results from contracture of both the GSC and soleus and a lengthening of both muscles may be required. More severe equinus deformity requires lengthening of the Achilles tendon that can be performed either open or percutaneous. In severe equinus contractures, additional procedures may be required, such as release of the plantar fascia to a correct forefoot equinus deformity, TA shortening to address the overlengthened TA, and toe flexor lengthenings to correct lesser toe deformities.[19,46]

## PES PLANOVALGUS

The planovalgus foot (flatfoot) is a variable, multiplanar deformity that is more commonly seen in spastic diplegia and spastic quadriplegia, than in children with hemiplegia. The deformity spectrum includes various degrees of hindfoot valgus, collapse of the medial longitudinal arch, midfoot breaching, convexity of the medial border of the foot, and forefoot abduction and secondary supination. Dorsolateral talonavicular joint subluxation can make bracing difficult and lead to skin callosities, breakdown, and pain overlying the uncovered head of the talus. Weight-bearing lateral radiographs of the foot demonstrate increased vertical tilting of the talus and decreased pitch of the os calcis.

Valgus deformity is primarily result of abnormal foot and ankle biomechanics, and to some extent dynamic muscle imbalance. Tibialis posterior deficiency may occur in patients with ambulatory CP (GMFCS I, II, and III). Peroneal overactivity may occur in nonambulatory children (GMFCS IV and V) and those with dystonia. Adaptive shortening of the GSC and the peroneal brevis may occur and GSC recession and peroneus brevis lengthening may be necessary to improve segmental joint alignment. Without foot correction surgery, planovalgus deformity progression may occur in ambulatory children with functional levels GMFCS II and III at highest risk.[47] The severity of the deformity is assessed by physical examination and radiographs. Gait analysis and pedobarography can be informative in the ambulatory child but are usually not necessary. Severe or longstanding deformity may be associated with hallux valgus, ankle valgus, external tibial torsion, and hip and knee flexion deformities (**Figs. 2A–C**).

In children with GMFCS levels I to III, planovalgus deformity may compromise gait by causing lever arm dysfunction.[48] Valgus malalignment of the hindfoot produces a malrotated lever-arm dysfunction by shortening the foot lever because of the externally rotated or abducted forefoot.[49,50] Midfoot breakdown and external tibial torsion contribute to deficiency in plantar flexion/knee extension coupling and often result in a crouch gait. Surgery in ambulatory patients with CP is indicated to relieve pain and

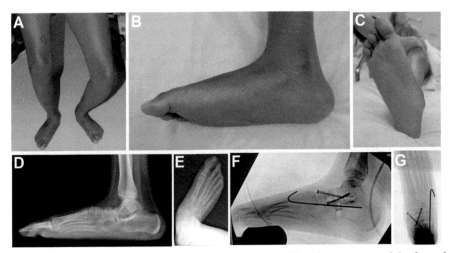

**Fig. 2.** Correction moderate planovalgus deformity. (*A–C*) Clinical appearance of the feet of an 11-year-old male with athetoid type CP, GMFCS level III, showing crouch gait and plano-valgus feet. (*D, E*) Weight-bearing AP and lateral (respectively) preoperative radiographs of the right foot demonstrating planovalgus malalignment. (*F, G*) Lateral and AP (respectively) intraoperative fluoroscopic radiographs of the foot following right calcaneal lengthening osteotomy and talonavicular fusion.

improve gait efficiency by addressing deformities causing lever arm dysfunction, especially when refractory to bracing. In general, surgical correction should preserve joint motion and correct all aspects of the lower limb deformity. Multiple surgical procedures have been described that reliably improve stance phase stability and functional ambulation. Those commonly used will be discussed (**Table 2**).

Perhaps the most well-described skeletal surgery for pes valgus is a lateral column lengthening first described by Evans[51] and popularized by Mosca.[52] Lateral column lengthening procedures equalize the lengths of the lateral column and medial column of the foot. They may be performed at the neck of the calcaneus, through the calcaneal cuboid joint, or in the body of the cuboid. The calcaneal lengthening osteotomy (CLO) allows for correction of all 3 segments of the foot.[53] The CLO is performed with an osteotomy at the anterior process of the os calcis and insertion of bone graft (usually iliac crest allograft). This procedure is recommended for flexible flat feet in children with GMFCS levels I and II. Lengthening of the peroneus brevis may also be required to retain the muscle and maximize graft size. Alternatively, correction can also be obtained with a medial calcaneal sliding osteotomy,[54] or calcaneo-cuboid-cuneiform osteotomies.[55] Arthroereisis performed with an assortment of available devices can have a high failure rate in children with severe CP and is generally not recommended in this population.[56,57] The authors have limited experience with the use of this technique. In the adolescent (older than 12 years) with moderate to severe deformity, a lateral lengthening-fusion may be performed through the calcaneocuboid joint. Plate fixation is often required as well as prolonged use of an AFO as graft incorporation can be slow.[58]

Once lateral column length is restored, the medial column should be assessed for shortening. Persistent forefoot abduction (midfoot break) and talonavicular subluxation after a CLO can be addressed with talonavicular arthrodesis. This concomitant procedure can reduce the risk of recurrent valgus.[59] Patients with GMFCS level III

**Table 2**
**Surgical bony procedures for planovalgus deformity**

| GMFCS | Procedure | Deformity Severity | Advantages/Disadvantages |
|---|---|---|---|
| Levels I–III | Calcaneal lengthening osteotomy | Mild | • Correction of all components of the deformity (hindfoot valgus, eversion, and forefoot abduction)<br>• Preserves joint motion<br>• Requires bone graft (usually allograft) |
| | Calcaneal medial sliding osteotomy | Mild | • Does not require bone graft<br>• Preserves joint motion |
| | Calcaneo-cuboid-cuneiform osteotomies | Mild<br>Mild to moderate forefoot adductus | • Addresses multiple components of flatfoot deformity<br>• Preserves joint motion |
| | Calcaneocuboid lengthening fusion | Mild to moderate<br>Severe forefoot adductus with short lateral column | • Limits joint motion<br>• Requires bone graft |
| Level III–V | Lateral column lengthening + TN arthrodesis | Moderate to severe | • Limits joint motion |
| | Extraarticular subtalar fusion ± TN arthrodesis | Moderate to severe | • Limits joint motion<br>• Requires bone graft |
| | Triple arthrodesis | Severe | • Severely limits hindfoot motion; should be used primarily in GMFCS IV and V<br>• Technically demanding (requires bone grafting of the sinus tarsi and lateral column with internal fixation)<br>• Requires bone graft |

| Additional Surgical Procedures | |
|---|---|
| **Deformity** | **Procedure** |
| Medial column collapse | • Posterior tibial tendon advancement with TN joint capsulorrhaphy<br>• Medial column stabilization with talonavicular arthrodesis |
| Supination of the first ray or sagittal plane hypermobility | • Plantar flexion osteotomy of the first metatarsal (do not perform if the physis is open)<br>• Plantar flexion osteotomy of the medial cuneiform |
| Ankle valgus | • Medial hemi-epiphysiodesis of the distal tibia (perform only if significant growth remains; countersink screw head to prevent skin irritation by an AFO or shoe)<br>• Supramalleolar osteotomy |
| External tibial torsion<br>Ankle plantar flexion | • Tibia ± fibula supramalleolar derotation osteotomy<br>• GSC recession |

*Abbreviation:* TN, talonavicular.

and obligate brace wearers may also need medial column stabilization at the time of lateral column lengthening surgery.[54,60,61] In milder cases, the medial column is stabilized with medial reefing (talonavicular joint capsulorrhaphy) and posterior tibial tendon advancement to reduce the risk of postoperative midfoot break. All the metatarsal heads should be parallel when the foot is inspected from the toes. Any persistent supination of the first ray, or hypermobility of the great toe metatarsal in the sagittal plane, following the lateral column lengthening should be concurrently addressed with a plantarflexion osteotomy of the medial cuneiform or the base of the first metatarsal. Next, the extremity must be examined for external tibial torsion, ankle valgus, and ankle plantar flexion malalignment. External tibial torsion can be corrected by supramalleolar osteotomy of the tibia.[62–64] Concomitant ankle valgus deformity can be addressed by medial malleolar screw epiphysiodesis if there is adequate growth remaining or by supramalleolar tibial osteotomy in the skeletally mature patient.[65] Lastly, ankle plantarflexion contracture should be corrected with a gastrocnemius recession or Achilles tendon lengthening. Failure to correct all deformities can lead to relapse and recurrent planovalgus deformity (see **Figs. 2**D–G).

For GMFCS levels III and IV with moderate to severe deformity that limits standing ability, surgical recommendations include combined calcaneocuboid and talonavicular fusion and occasionally an extraarticular subtalar fusion with bone graft.[58,66,67] For GMFCS levels IV and V, as well as children with dystonia, with severe subtalar hindfoot valgus, a triple arthrodesis may be required. Surgery is indicated in patients with brace/shoe wear intolerance and compromised wheelchair sitting. Triple arthrodesis can occasionally be combined with a calcaneocuboid lengthening fusion to minimize the need for medial column shortening.[68]

## EQUINOVARUS

Equinovarus deformity is a complex and variable deformity that is more common in children with spastic hemiplegia and quadriplegia than diplegia. Segmental malalignment involves hindfoot varus, midfoot adduction, forefoot pronation, ankle equinus, and occasionally forefoot cavus (equinocavovarus). The deformity results from dynamic muscle imbalance, with the foot invertors and plantar flexors overpowering the evertors. Over time, the foot stiffens and function is compromised by impaired shock absorption and a decreased weight-bearing area. Pain, calluses, and stress fractures can occur over the lateral aspect of the forefoot and compromise shoe wear, bracing, and mobility. Indications for surgery include older children who are refractory to botulinum toxin injection and serial casting, have foot pain, or have brace or shoe wear intolerance. In the ambulatory child, fixed versus flexible deformity of the hindfoot can be identified on examination by the modified Coleman block test, whereby a 2.5 cm block is placed under the lateral 2 to 3 metatarsal heads rather than the entire lateral column of the foot.[69]

For flexible deformities, soft-tissue surgery is needed to rebalance the deforming muscle forces using a combination of soft-tissue releases, tendon transfers, and/or lengthenings. There is consensus that overactive or inappropriately firing muscles should be lengthened or transferred. However, there is controversy regarding the best procedure (or combination of procedures) that appropriately balances the foot and minimizes the risk of recurrent varus deformity and valgus overcorrection with continued growth of the child. Determining the best method to assess the relative contributions of TA and TP to the equinovarus foot is debated. Physical examination, radiographs, gait analysis, dynamic EMG, and pedobarography are all important in assessing soft-tissue and skeletal deformities and help guide surgical management. Overactivity of the TA can be determined on physical examination with a positive confusion test.[70] EMG analysis has revealed that varus deformity can be due to overactivity of the TA, TP, or both muscles.[71] Davids and colleagues have recommended performing a split transfer of TA (SPLATT) when there is ankle dorsiflexion in midstance; and a split transfer of the PT (SPOTT) when dynamic EMG demonstrates that the timing of PT corresponds with the presence of varus malalignment during specific phases of the gait.[12]

Typically, the muscles that demonstrate overactivity during gait on EMG should be addressed. TA overactivity is commonly treated with an SPLATT. The lateral hemitendon of TA is transferred either to the cuboid or base of the fifth metatarsal, or to the peroneus brevis.[72-74] When there is concurrent TP overactivity, intramuscular lengthening of TP is combined with SPLATT. Z-lengthening of the TP should be undertaken in adolescents and adults with more severe or rigid deformities. Most patients with hemiplegia require an SPLATT, combined with a muscle lengthening of the TP and GSC, also known as a Rancho procedure. TP lengthenings should be avoided in patients with spastic diplegia because of the greater risk of overcorrection. SPLATT should be avoided in patients with a "drop foot" gait that occurs during the swing phase of gait, nonambulators, as well as in patients with a fixed bony deformity. Overall, favorable results can be expected following SPLATT with better outcomes in children with spastic hemiplegia than in children with spastic diplegia and quadriplegia.[75,76]

Isolated TP overactivity can be managed by either an intramuscular lengthening or split transfer of the TP tendon. A split transfer is usually preferred as it does not result in loss of muscle power. The hemi-tendon is usually routed around the lateral malleolus and secured to the peroneus brevis. After surgery is performed to rebalance the TA and/or TP, the ankle should be reassessed for any plantar flexion deformity. If indicated, a GSC recession is preferred to an Achilles tendon lengthening to avoid overcorrection. Other factors that should be considered when contemplating such tendon transfer include the geographic pattern of CP, age at operation, and preoperative status of ambulation. Chang and colleagues reported that children with spastic hemiplegia do well regardless of age, whereas children with diplegia and quadriplegia who are younger than 8 years or are not capable of community ambulation are at risk for poor outcomes with operative treatment.[77]

Severe equinovarus deformity and those with skeletal deformity often require bony procedures. Soft-tissue balancing should be performed either before or with bony surgery. Unlike planovalgus foot correction with lateral column lengthening procedures, there is no single osteotomy that can adequately achieve multisegmental correction. Corrective osteotomies for equinovarus improve gross alignment but create secondary deformities to compensate for segmental malalignment rather than obtaining correction at or near the site of deformity. Hindfoot varus malalignment may be corrected by a lateral calcaneal slide or a laterally based closing wedge osteotomy, or a combination of both techniques.[78,79] Residual midfoot adductus and rigid supination may be corrected with a dorsolateral-based closing wedge cuboid osteotomy and a medial opening wedge osteotomy of the medial cuneiform. Residual forefoot cavus and inversion may be corrected with a dorsally based closing wedge osteotomy of the medial cuneiform or first proximal metatarsal (when the proximal physis has closed). In more severe cavus deformity, a dorsiflexion Lapidus procedure may be required to achieve optimal foot alignment. Tendon transfers (often split tendon transfers) to correct coexisting dynamic muscle imbalance should be performed following bony surgery to ensure appropriate balancing of the soft tissues. Triple arthrodesis may be required for more severe deformities. The surgeon often begins with first correcting hindfoot varus, then midfoot supination, and finally forefoot inversion by arthrodesis of the subtalar joint, calcaneocuboid joint, and talonavicular joint, respectively.

## HALLUX VALGUS AND DORSAL BUNIONS

First metatarsophalangeal (MTP) deformities are common in patients with CP and may become severe enough to warrant surgical intervention. Symptomatic toe deformities typically develop in the adolescents and teenagers in 2 distinct populations of patients with CP.[80] Hallux valgus frequently occurs in older children with predominantly spastic motor disorder, GMFCS levels II and III, who have had prior SEMLS to improve gait function. In contrast, dorsal bunion deformity usually occurs in patients with dystonia or spastic dystonia, GMFCS levels IV and V, with a high prevalence of concomitant hip displacement and spinal deformity.

Hallux valgus deformity may cause pain and callosities on the medial side of the first MTP joint, affect shoe wear or the use of orthotics, cause poor foot hygiene (overlapping or underlapping of the great and second toes), nail infection, gait dysfunction, and may appear unsightly, especially for teenage girls. Surgical treatment for hallux valgus should be considered for patients with a fixed deformity and continued pain after attempts at conservative management, including a wide shoe and orthotic modification. Hallux valgus surgery should be performed in conjunction with the treatment of other segmental malalignments of the foot, most commonly planovalgus, and dynamic gait deviation of the lower extremities (**Figs. 3**A–B).[81] Because of high recurrence rates in a patient with CP, correction is usually performed with a first MTP arthrodesis. Soft-tissue surgery alone leads to poor outcomes. Soft-tissue surgery in combination with first metatarsal osteotomy, proximal phalanx osteotomy, and correction of midfoot and hindfoot segmental malalignment may lead to good results. This approach preserves mobility at the MTP joint, which is important for push-off for heel-to-toe gait and is a viable surgical option in patients with GMFCS levels I to III with mild deformities and no degenerative arthritis of the MTP joint.[81,82] However, to date, there is little data on the long-term success of nonfusion surgery in patients with CP.

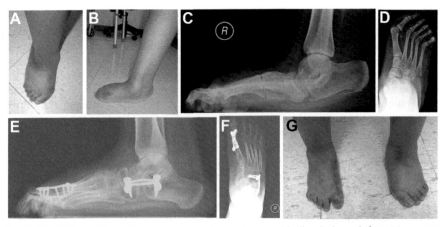

**Fig. 3.** (*A, B*) Correction of severe equinoplanovalgus and hallux halgus deformities. A 12-year-old female with spastic diplegia CP, GMFCS level III, with painful feet interfering with ambulation and use of orthoses. (*C, D*) AP and lateral (respectively) preoperative weight-bearing radiographs of the right foot demonstrating equinoplanovalgus malalignment. (*E, F*) 4 months postoperative weight-bearing AP and lateral radiographs following a gastrocnemius recession, calcaneocuboid lengthening arthrodesis, and first MTP arthrodesis demonstrating improved alignment of the foot, including the talonavicular joint. (*G*) Clinical appearance of the feet after surgical correction on the right.

Dorsal bunion (hallux flexus) is characterized by elevation of the first ray and plantar-flexion of the first MTP joint. It is less common than hallux valgus and usually remains asymptomatic until midteens.[80] It occurs in adolescents with spastic-dystonia but may also occur iatrogenically after pes valgus correction. Patients with dorsal bunion often present with pain and skin breakdown over the dorsum of the first MTP joint. In patients who fail nonoperative treatment such as shoe modifications and orthosis, surgical management with a first MTP joint fusion is the preferred treatment.

## SUMMARY

Foot deformities in children with CP are a consequence of dynamic muscle imbalance and abnormal biomechanics over time and are often seen in both ambulatory and non-ambulatory patients. These deformities may disrupt shock absorption and lever function of the foot during stance phase in the ambulatory patient. Surgical correction of foot deformities is performed to improve lever function of the foot by optimizing foot shape and improving shock absorption function by optimizing intrasegmental and intersegmental alignment. It is important to address all pathologic segmental malalignments at the time of surgery by realigning the joints with soft-tissue releases, correcting bony deformities, and finally appropriate muscle balancing. When necessary, muscle fascia and intramuscular lengthening are favored over muscle releases and tendon lengthening, and osteotomy is preferred over arthrodesis to restore foot skeletal segmental alignment. Foot deformity correction should be performed as part of multilevel surgery to improve gait function in children with CP.

## CLINICS CARE POINTS

---

- Treatment should be tailored to each individual child.
- The principle of "surgical dosing" is a critical factor in selecting the appropriate procedure.
- Foot deformity correction should be performed as part of multilevel surgery to improve gait function in children with CP.

---

## DISCLOSURE

The authors have nothing to disclose.

## REFERENCES

1. Howard J, Soo B, Graham HK, et al. Cerebral palsy in Victoria: motor types, topography and gross motor function. J Pediatr Child Health 2005;41:479–83.
2. Shore BJ, Thomason SM, Reid S, et al. Cerebral palsy. In: Weinstein SL, Flynn JM, Crawford H, editors. Lovell and winter's pediatric orthopaedics. 8th edition. Philadelphia: Wolters Kluwer Health/Lippincott Williams & Wilkins; 2020. p. 509–50.
3. Rosenbaum P, Paneth N, Leviton A, et al. A report: the definition and classification of cerebral palsy April 2006. Dev Med Child Neurol Suppl 2007;109:8–14.
4. O'Connell PA, D'Souza L, Dudeney S, et al. Foot deformities in children with cerebral palsy. J Pediatr Orthop 1998;18(6):743–7.
5. Graham HK, Rosenbaum P, Paneth N, et al. Cerebral palsy. Nat Rev Dis Primers 2016;7(2):15082.

6. Palisano R, Rosenbaum P, Walter S, et al. Development and reliability of a system to classify gross motor function in children with cerebral palsy. Dev Med Child Neurol 1997;39(4):214–23.

7. Rosenbaum PL, Palisano RJ, Bartlett DJ, et al. Development of the gross motor function classification system for cerebral palsy. Dev Med Child Neurol 2008; 50(4):249–53.

8. Rosenbaum PL, Walter SD, Hanna SE, et al. Prognosis for gross motor function in cerebral palsy: creation of motor development curves. JAMA 2002;288(11): 1357–63.

9. Hanna SE, Rosenbaum PL, Bartlett DJ, et al. Stability and decline in gross motor function among children and youth with cerebral palsy aged 2 to 21 years. Dev Med Child Neurol 2009;51(4):295–302.

10. Johnson DC, Damiano DL, Abel MF. The evolution of gait in childhood and adolescent cerebral palsy. J Pediatr Orthop 1997;17(3):392–6.

11. Chambers HG, Chambers RC. Introduction to the cerebral palsies. In: Nowicki PD, editor. Orthopedic care of patients with cerebral palsy. Switzerland: Springer; 2020. p. 7–11.

12. Graham HK, Thomason P, Willoughby K, et al. Musculoskeletal pathology in cerebral palsy: a classification system and reliability study. Children (Basel) 2021; 23(3):252.

13. Sutherland DH, Olshen R, Cooper L, et al. The development of mature gait. J Bone Joint Surg Am 1980;62(3):336–53.

14. Graham HK, Selber P. Musculoskeletal aspects of cerebral palsy. J Bone J Surg Br 2003;85(2):157–66.

15. Rattey TE, Leahey L, Hyndman J, et al. Recurrence after Achilles tendon lengthening in cerebral palsy. J Pediatr Orthop 1993;13(2):184–7.

16. Borton DC, Walker K, Pirpiris M, et al. Isolated calf lengthening in cerebral palsy. Outcome analysis of risk factors. J Bone Joint Surg Br 2001;83(3):364–70.

17. Chung CY, Sung KH, Lee KM, et al. Recurrence of equinus foot deformity after tendo-achilles lengthening in patients with cerebral palsy. J Pediatr Orthop 2015;35(4):419–25.

18. Davids JR. The foot and ankle in cerebral palsy. Orthop Clin North Am 2010; 41(4):579–93.

19. Davids JR, Ounpuu S, DeLuca PA, et al. Optimization of walking ability of children with cerebral palsy. Instr Course Lect 2004;53:511–22.

20. Blair E. Epidemiology of the cerebral palsies. Orthop Clin North Am 2010;41(4): 441–55.

21. Bax M, Tydeman C, Flodmark O. Clinical and MRI correlates of cerebral palsy: the European cerebral palsy study. JAMA 2006;296:1602–8.

22. Sanger TD, Delgado MR, Gaebler-Spira D, et al. Task Force on Childhood Motor Disorders. Classification and definition of disorders causing hypertonia in childhood. Pediatrics 2003;111:e89–97.

23. Blumetti FC, Wu JCN, Barzi F, et al. Orthopaedic surgery in dystonic cerebral palsy. J Pediatr Orthop 2019;39(4):209–16.

24. Fulford GE. Surgical management of ankle and foot deformities in cerebral palsy. Clin Orthop Relat Res 1990;253:55–61.

25. Sees JP, Miller F. Overview of foot deformity management in children with cerebral palsy. J Child Orthop 2013;7(5):373–7.

26. Davids JR, Gibson TW, Pugh LI. Quantitative segmental analysis of weight-bearing radiographs of the foot and ankle for children: normal alignment. J Pediatr Orthop 2005;25(6):769–76.

27. White H, Augsburger S. Gait evaluation for patients with cerebral palsy. In: Nowicki PD, editor. Orthopedic care of patients with cerebral palsy. Switzerland: Springer; 2020. p. 51–76.

28. Scott AC, Scarborough N. The use of dynamic EMG in predicting the outcome of split posterior tibial tendon transfers in spastic hemiplegia. J Pediatr Orthop 2006;26(6):777–80.

29. Hoffer MM, Barakat G, Koffman M. 10-year follow-up of split anterior tibial tendon transfer in cerebral palsied patients with spastic equinovarus deformity. J Pediatr Orthop 1985;5(4):432–4.

30. Chang CH, Miller F, Schuyler J. Dynamic pedobarograph in evaluation of varus and valgus foot deformities. J Pediatr Orthop 2002;22(6):813–8.

31. Mosca VS. The child's foot: principles of management. J Pediatr Orthop 1998; 18(3):281–2.

32. Pierz M, Shrader W. Multilevel orthopedic surgery for patients with cerebral palsy. In: Nowicki PD, editor. Orthopedic care of patients with cerebral palsy. Switzerland: Springer; 2020. p. 77–92.

33. Thomason P, Selber P, Graham HK. Single Event Multilevel Surgery in children with bilateral spastic cerebral palsy: a 5 year prospective cohort study. Gait Posture 2013;37(1):23–8.

34. Bischof FM. Single event multilevel surgery in cerebral palsy: a review of the literature. SA Orthop J 2010;9(1):30–3.

35. Švehlík M, Steinwender G, Lehmann T, et al. Predictors of outcome after single-event multilevel surgery in children with cerebral palsy: a retrospective ten-year follow-up study. Bone Joint J 2016;98-B(2):278–81.

36. Graham HK, Natrass GR, Selber PR. Re: kinematic and kinetic evaluation of the ankle joint before and after tendo Achilles lengthening in patients with spastic diplegia –. J Pediatr Orthop 2005;25:479–83.

37. Firth GB, McMullan M, Chin T, et al. Lengthening of the gastrocnemius-soleus complex: an anatomical and biomechanical study in human cadavers. J Bone Joint Surg Am 2013;95(16):1489–96.

38. Joo SY, Knowtharapu DN, Rogers KJ, et al. Recurrence after surgery for equinus foot deformity in children with cerebral palsy: assessment of predisposing factors for recurrence in a long-term follow-up study. J Child Orthop 2011;5(4):289–96.

39. Olney BW, Williams PF, Menelaus MB. Treatment of spastic equinus by aponeurosis lengthening. J Pediatr Orthop 1988;8(4):422–5.

40. Rodda JM, Graham HK, Nattrass GR, et al. Correction of severe crouch gait in patients with spastic diplegia with use of multilevel orthopaedic surgery. J Bone Joint Surg Am 2006;88(12):2653–64.

41. Graham K. Cerebral palsy. In: McCarthy JJ, Drennan JC, editors. Drennan's the child's foot & ankle. 2nd edition. Philadelphia: Lippincott Williams & Wilkins; 2010. p. 188–218.

42. Rodda JM, Graham HK, Carson L, et al. Sagittal gait patterns in spastic diplegia. J Bone Joint Surg Br 2004;86(2):251–8.

43. Wren TA, Cheatwood AP, Rethlefsen SA, et al. Achilles tendon length and medial gastrocnemius architecture in children with cerebral palsy and equinus gait. J Pediatr Orthop 2010;30(5):479–84.

44. Firth GB, Passmore E, Sangeux M, et al. Multilevel surgery for equinus gait in children with spastic diplegic cerebral palsy: medium-term follow-up with gait analysis. J Bone Joint Surg Am 2013;95(10):931–8.

45. Dietz FR, Albright JC, Dolan L. Medium-term follow-up of Achilles tendon lengthening in the treatment of ankle equinus in cerebral palsy. Iowa Orthop J 2006;26: 27–32.
46. Rutz E, Baker R, Tirosh O, et al. Tibialis anterior tendon shortening in combination with Achilles tendon lengthening in spastic equinus in cerebral palsy. Gait Posture 2011;33(2):152–7.
47. Min JJ, Kwon SS, Sung KH, et al. Progression of planovalgus deformity in patients with cerebral palsy. BMC Musculoskelet Disord 2020;21(1):141.
48. Theologis T. Lever arm dysfunction in cerebral palsy gait. J Child Orthop 2013; 7(5):379–82.
49. Kalkman BM, Bar-On L, Cenni F, et al. Achilles tendon moment arm length is smaller in children with cerebral palsy than in typically developing children. J Biomech 2017;56:48–54.
50. Novacheck TF, Gage JR. Orthopedic management of spasticity in cerebral palsy. Childs Nerv Syst 2007;23(9):1015–31.
51. Evans D. Calcaneo-valgus deformity. J Bone Joint Surg Br 1975;57(3):270–8.
52. Mosca VS. Calcaneal lengthening for valgus deformity of the hindfoot. Results in children who had severe, symptomatic flatfoot and skewfoot. J Bone Joint Surg Am 1995;77(4):500–12.
53. Sangeorzan BJ, Mosca V, Hansen ST Jr. Effect of calcaneal lengthening on relationships among the hindfoot, midfoot, and forefoot. Foot Ankle 1993;14(3): 136–41.
54. Rethlefsen SA, Hanson AM, Wren TAL, et al. Calcaneal sliding osteotomy versus calcaneal lengthening osteotomy for valgus foot deformity correction in children with cerebral palsy. J Pediatr Orthop 2021;41(6):e433–8.
55. Moraleda L, Salcedo M, Bastrom TP, et al. Comparison of the calcaneo-cuboid-cuneiform osteotomies and the calcaneal lengthening osteotomy in the surgical treatment of symptomatic flexible flatfoot. J Pediatr Orthop 2012;32(8):821–9.
56. Smith PA, Millar EA, Sullivan RC. Sta-Peg arthroereisis for treatment of the plano-valgus foot in cerebral palsy. Clin Podiatr Med Surg 2000;17(3):459–69.
57. Sanchez AA, Rathjen KE, Mubarak SJ. Subtalar staple arthroereisis for planovalgus foot deformity in children with neuromuscular disease. J Pediatr Orthop 1999; 19(1):34–8.
58. Costici PF, Donati F, Russo R, et al. Double hindfoot arthrodesis technique for the treatment of severe equino-plano-valgus foot deformity in cerebral palsy: long-term results and radiological evaluation. J Pediatr Orthop B 2019;28(3):235–41.
59. Cho BC, Lee IH, Chung CY, et al. Undercorrection of planovalgus deformity after calcaneal lengthening in patients with cerebral palsy. J Pediatr Orthop B 2018; 27(3):206–13.
60. Goodbody C, Tedesco L, Vosseller JT, et al. Orthopedic foot and ankle surgery for patients with cerebral palsy. In: Nowicki PD, editor. Orthopedic care of patients with cerebral palsy. Switzerland: Springer; 2020. p. 171–92.
61. Huang CN, Wu KW, Huang SC, et al. Medial column stabilization improves the early result of calcaneal lengthening in children with cerebral palsy. J Pediatr Orthop B 2013;22(3):233–9.
62. Ryan DD, Rethlefsen SA, Skaggs DL, et al. Results of tibial rotational osteotomy without concomitant fibular osteotomy in children with cerebral palsy. J Pediatr Orthop 2005;25(1):84–8.
63. Selber P, Filho ER, Dallalana R, et al. Supramalleolar derotation osteotomy of the tibia, with T plate fixation. Technique and results in patients with neuromuscular disease. J Bone Joint Surg Br 2004;86(8):1170–5.

64. Sarikaya IA, Seker A, Erdal OA, et al. Minimally invasive plate osteosynthesis for tibial derotation osteotomies in children with cerebral palsy. Acta Orthop Traumatol Turc 2018;52(5):352–6.
65. Davids JR, Valadie AL, Ferguson RL, et al. Surgical management of ankle valgus in children: use of a transphyseal medial malleolar screw. J Pediatr Orthop 1997; 17(1):3–8.
66. Dogan A, Zorer G, Mumcuoglu EI, et al. A comparison of two different techniques in the surgical treatment of flexible pes planovalgus: calcaneal lengthening and extra-articular subtalar arthrodesis. J Pediatr Orthop B 2009;18(4):167–75.
67. Yoon HK, Park KB, Roh JY, et al. Extraarticular subtalar arthrodesis for pes planovalgus: an interim result of 50 feet in patients with spastic diplegia. Clin Orthop Surg 2010;2:13–21.
68. Horton GA, Olney BW. Triple arthrodesis with lateral column lengthening for treatment of severe planovalgus deformity. Foot Ankle Int 1995;16(7):395–400.
69. Mosca VS. Principles and management of pediatric foot and ankle deformities and Malformations. Philadelphia: Wolters Kluwer; 2014.
70. Davids JR, Holland WC, Sutherland DH. Significance of the confusion test in cerebral palsy. J Pediatr Orthop 1993;13(6):717–21.
71. Michlitsch MG, Rethlefsen SA, Kay RM. The contributions of anterior and posterior tibialis dysfunction to varus foot deformity in patients with cerebral palsy. J Bone Joint Surg Am 2006;88(8):1764–8.
72. Hosalkar H, Goebel J, Reddy S. Fixation techniques for split anterior tibialis transfer in spastic equinovarus feet. Clin Orthop Relat Res 2008;466(10):2500–6.
73. Gasse N, Luth T, Loisel F, et al. Fixation of split anterior tibialis tendon transfer by anchorage to the base of the 5th metatarsal bone. Orthop Traumatol Surg Res 2012;98(7):829–33.
74. Wong P, Fransch S, Gallagher C, et al. Split anterior tibialis tendon transfer to peroneus brevis for spastic equinovarus in children with hemiplegia. J Child Orthop 2021;15(3):279–90.
75. Vlachou M, Dimitriadis D. Split tendon transfers for the correction of spastic varus foot deformity: a case series study. J Foot Ankle Res 2010;3:28.
76. Lullo B, Nazareth A, Rethlefsen S, et al. Split tibialis anterior tendon transfer to the peroneus brevis or Tertius for the treatment of varus foot deformities in children with static encephalopathy: a retrospective case series. J Am Acad Orthop Surg Glob Res Rev 2020;4(5):e2000044.
77. Chang CH, Albarracin JP, Lipton GE, et al. Long-term follow-up of surgery for equinovarus foot deformity in children with cerebral palsy. J Pediatr Orthop 2002;22(6):792–9.
78. Cody EA, Kraszewski AP, Conti MS, et al. Lateralizing calcaneal osteotomies and their effect on calcaneal alignment: a three-dimensional digital model analysis. Foot Ankle Int 2018;39(8):970–7.
79. An TW, Michalski M, Jansson K, et al. Comparison of lateralizing calcaneal osteotomies for varus hindfoot correction. Foot Ankle Int 2018;39(10):1229–36.
80. van de Velde SK, Cashin M, Johari R, et al. Symptomatic hallux valgus and dorsal bunion in adolescents with cerebral palsy: clinical and biomechanical factors. Dev Med Child Neurol 2018;60(6):624–8.
81. Sarikaya IA, Seker A, Erdal OA, et al. Surgical correction of hallux valgus deformity in children with cerebral palsy. Acta Orthop Traumatol Turc 2018;52(3):174–8.
82. Bayhan IA, Kadhim M, Sees JP, et al. Hallux valgus deformity correction without fusion in children with cerebral palsy. J Pediatr Orthop B 2017;26(2):164–71.

# Pediatric Trauma

Gan Golshteyn, MS, DPM*, Anna Katsman, MD

## KEYWORDS

- Trauma • Dislocations • Fractures

## KEY POINTS

- Musculoskeletal injuries of the lower limb are frequent in pediatric patients and represent the most common cause of Emergency Department admissions.
- Routine plain film radiographs of the foot consisting of anteroposterior (AP), lateral, and oblique projections, and ankle AP, mortise, and lateral radiographs should be obtained of patients with persistent ankle pain, especially those who cannot bear weight.
- Salter-Harris classification the most commonly used fracture classification system utilized for pediatric fractures involving the physeal plates.

## INTRODUCTION

Musculoskeletal injuries of the lower limb are frequent in pediatric patients and represent the most common cause of emergency department admissions. It is estimated that 1 in 4 children sustain an unintentional injury that requires medical care each year.[1] Skeletal trauma in children differ from those injuries in adults, and hence the need to address it differently. Injuries of the growth plate account for 15% to 30% of all pediatric fractures and deserve special attention, and long-term follow-up is appropriate because of the increased risk of growth disturbances, angular deformity, and/or premature physeal closure.[2–4] Dislocations and ligamentous injuries are uncommon in the pediatric population, as the physes act as the weakest point, bearing the load for trauma.[2]

Acute sports-related injuries commonly involve the lower extremity, as the knee and ankle are the most frequently injured parts. Acute ankle sprains are the most common injuries of all sports, accounting for 15% of all reported acute, nonsevere injuries, while knee injuries are noted to be associated with severe injuries, accounting for 44.6% of all surgeries.[5,6] Nearly 25% of pediatric patients that present to the emergency department with lower extremity injuries involve a fracture, with phalanx fractures representing the most common physeal injury.[7–10] The tibia and fibular fractures account for 6.1% while ankle fractures account for 5% of the pediatric lower extremity trauma. Physeal fractures are common injuries in children and adolescents participating in

The Pediatric Orthopedic Center, 218 Ridgedale Ave #101, Cedar Knolls, NJ 07927, USA
* Corresponding author. 6145 N. Thesta Street, Fresno, CA 93710.
*E-mail address:* gan.golshteyn@gmail.com

Clin Podiatr Med Surg 39 (2022) 57–71
https://doi.org/10.1016/j.cpm.2021.08.001      **podiatric.theclinics.com**

contact sports, which may lead to growth disturbances and cause limb length discrepancy.

## MANAGEMENT OF PEDIATRIC TRAUMA

Pediatric injuries result in more deaths in children and young adolescents than all other causes combined.[11,12] It is estimated that 1 in 4 children sustain an unintentional injury that requires medical attention each year.[1] The leading cause of death in children aged 1 to 14 years is accidental trauma, and skeletal trauma accounts for 10% to 15% of all childhood injuries with roughly 15% to 30% of these representing physeal injuries.[10] Therefore, understanding pediatric trauma in efforts to improve outcomes for the injured child requires an approach that is vital to the health care system. It has been demonstrated that younger and more seriously injured children have better outcomes once treated at a trauma center within a children's hospital or at a trauma center that integrates pediatric and adult trauma.[13,14] The overall ratio of boys to girls who sustain a single, isolated pediatric fracture is 2.7:1.[10] The peak incidence of fractures in pediatric males occurs at the age of 16 years, with an incidence of 450 per 10,000/y; pediatric female fractures occur at an average age of 12 years with a peak incidence of 250 per 10,000/y.[10] Each child that presents to the emergency department requires special consideration to his/her own injury. Examples of some of the issues that are unique to children include diagnostic radiation exposure, family presence during resuscitation, the availability of child life specialists, fluid and electrolyte management, and blood transfusions.[15] It is imperative for pediatric trauma centers to implement evidence-based multispecialty protocols for the perimanagement of the injured child, especially through the postdischarge and rehabilitation phases, in order for the child to resume active daily living.

## IMAGING

Pediatric foot and ankle fractures pose a diagnostic challenge to foot and ankle physicians, especially in the absence of obvious plain film radiographic findings. One must have thorough knowledge of the anatomy and significance of accessory ossicles (bones) that may be present on radiographic findings in the foot and ankle, as well as disorders of the growing skeleton that may be helpful in diagnosis and managing the injured extremity. The physician should be aware of accessory ossicles at the

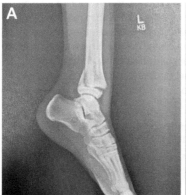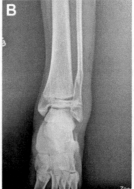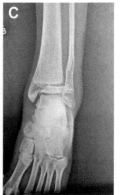

**Fig. 1.** (A–C) Pediatric foot and ankle fracture poses.

ankle joint, which are estimated at 5.2% at each of the malleoli.[16] The presence of an ossicle rather than a fracture is noted by a smooth cortical edge, the absence of soft tissue swelling near the malleoli, and no periosteal reaction on repeat plain film radiographs.[16] Infants and young children undergo routine imaging studies to evaluate a wide variety of congenital and acquired disorders.[17] Routine plain film radiographs of the foot consisting of anteroposterior (AP), lateral, and oblique projections and ankle AP, mortise, and lateral radiographs should be obtained of patients with persistent ankle pain, especially those who cannot bear weight.[17,18] When taking images of a pediatric patient, the physician and radiology technician must take into account the patient's comfort, age, level of anxiety, and the size of the patient to decrease radiation with appropriate imaging exposure[18] (**Fig. 1**).

Magnetic resonance imaging (MRI) provides excellent diagnostic ability and visualization of anatomic detail and information regarding cartilaginous, vasculature, and tendinous injuries, as well as soft-tissue masses and fracture lines.[17,19,20] Computed tomography (CT) imaging can be invaluable in surgical planning, especially injuries involving intra-articular fractures because it offers enhanced delineation of fracture alignment and displacement.[17,18] However, CT imaging exposes the patient to higher radiation than MRI and does not adequately define the nonossified portions of the bones, which should be taken into account in pediatric trauma. However, MRI has the capability of demonstrating early vascular and cartilaginous changes and visualizing any soft-tissue injury and subsequent hematoma in the injured patient.[21–24] There is a growing concern about the long-term risks of radiation delivery in the pediatric population. Kern and colleagues performed a retrospective study of 163 patients (females, aged 0.5–19 years; males aged 3.1–19 years) who sustained an orthopedic extremity injury that required a CT scan in the supine position.[25] They concluded that lower extremity CT scans were more frequent (124/163, 76%) than upper extremity CT scans and had a higher radiation dose overall. The study noted that variability in positioning and delineation of scout contributed to variation in radiation exposure of extremity and adjacent body area. Improved localization and consistent position can lower radiation exposure in children under a necessary CT scan.[25]

## TIBIA AND FIBULA
### Anatomy of the Tibia

The tibia is a triangular shape with an anteriorly directed apex that broadens gradually distally. The anteromedial surface of the tibia, which is immediately subcutaneous and easily palpable, has no muscular or ligamentous attachments distal to the pes anserinus.[19] The tibial flare distally primarily leads to cancellous bone and a thin cortical shell. The anterolateral surface of the tibia is the site of many muscular attachments and forms the medial wall of the anterior compartment of the leg. The extensor hallucis longus muscle, tibialis anterior muscle, and the neurovascular bundle are adjacent to this surface.[19] Posteriorly, the tibia has a large soft-tissue envelope with attachments from the semimembranosus muscle, popliteus muscle, tibialis posterior muscle, and flexor digitorum longus muscle. The tibia has been modeled as taking an axial force during gait that is up to 4.7 times the bodyweight. Its bending moment in the sagittal plane in the late stance phase is up to 71.6 times the bodyweight times millimeter.[26,27]

The fibula is subcutaneous proximally and supports the attachments from the lateral collateral ligament and the biceps femoris muscle to the fibular head.[19] The fibular head is an irregular quadrate presenting above a flattened articular surface with a corresponding surface on the lateral condyle of the tibial. The common peroneal nerve courses posterior to anterior over the distal portion of the fibular head, where it then divides into the superficial peroneal and deep peroneal branches.[19] The fibula is surrounded by a large soft-tissue envelope that is composed primarily of muscular attachments, consisting of the peroneus brevis and peroneus longus muscle. The lateral malleolus, which is a common site of pediatric fractures due to the presence of the physis, articulates with the distal tibia and talus and provides significant stability to the ankle joint.[19] A thick oblique-oriented interosseous membrane supports the articulation between the fibula and tibia, running from the anteromedial border of the fibula to the lateral crest of the tibia.

The tibia has three ossification centers. The tibial diaphysis ossifies at 7 weeks of gestation, the proximal tibial epiphysis appears a few months after birth, and the distal tibial epiphysis develops in the second year of life.[19] The fibular diaphysis ossifies at 8 weeks of gestation, and the proximal secondary center of ossification of the fibula appears at 4 years of age as the distal fibular epiphysis appears at 2 years of age.[19] Closure of the proximal tibial and fibular physis occurs between 16 and 18 years of age, and the distal tibial and fibular physis usually close at age 16 years. Physeal closure in females usually occurs before males with the onset of menstruation. The medial malleolus and tibial tubercle may present as separate ossification centers and should be carefully evaluated to not be confused with a fracture. In contrast to other physeal plates in long bones, tibial physeal closure occurs slowly and eccentrically, starting around the Poland hump and moving anteromedially, posterolaterally, and finally anterolaterally. The distal tibial physis provides approximately 40% of the growth of the tibia and 17% of the lower extremity, equating to 3-4 mm of growth per year in childhood. The growth of the distal tibia occurs proportionately to the proximal tibia in younger pediatric patients; however, during the adolescent years, the proximal tibia growth becomes more rapid as distal tibial growth tapers off.[28]

The major blood supply to the tibia arises from three main arteries[5]: the nutrient artery as a branch of the posterior tibial artery[29]; the epiphyseal vessels; and[6] the periosteal vessels.[10,19,30] The course of the nutrient artery of the human tibia was described in detail by Crock, who noted that the nutrient artery arises from the anterior aspect of the posterior tibial artery, very close to the origin of the popliteal artery.[31,32] The nutrient artery enters the posterior aspect of the proximal portion of the tibia and courses proximally and distally to anastomose with the metaphyseal endosteal vessels.[19] The outer two-third of the tibial diaphysis is supplied by the anastomosing periosteal vessels, and the inner two-third of the tibial diaphysis is supplied by the nutrient artery.[31] A fracture of the tibia would result in recruitment of the peripheral vessels to supply the majority of blood flow to the tibial cortex for revascularization of the necrotic, fractured area[31–33]

## FRACTURES OF THE TIBIA AND FIBULA

Pediatric tibial fractures represent 15% of pediatric fractures and are noted to be the third most common pediatric long bone fractures, after forearm and femoral fractures, with an average age of occurrence of 8 years.[10] The distal tibial epiphysis is the second most common site of fracture that involves the epiphyseal plate.[34,35] Of all physeal injuries, fractures of the distal tibial physis are associated with one of the highest rates of complications, including premature physeal closure, angular deformity, bar formation, and articular incongruity, pending the degree of force applied to the bone.[28,36,37] The physeal plate contains 4 zones, extending from the epiphysis to the metaphysis: (1) the proliferative zone; (2) the hypertrophic zone; (3) the reserve zone; and (4) the provisional calcification zone. Fractures involving the physis typically occur through the hypertrophic zone, which contains the largest cells and less extracellular matrix than the other physeal zones.[28] In return, this preserves the reserve zone of the physeal plate, which is located on the epiphyseal side of the fracture and contains progenitor cells for physeal growth.[28,38]

A pediatric patient with an ankle fracture should be examined appropriately according to the Advanced Trauma Life Support principles, and any life-threatening injuries should be assessed for open fractures, neurovascular compromise, and compartment syndrome.[39] The entire limb should be examined, and the overlying skin should be examined for bruises, ecchymosis, and tenting, which would require immediate closed reduction maneuver urgently.

## SALTER-HARRIS CLASSIFICATION OF PEDIATRIC PHYSEAL FRACTURES

Fractures involving the epiphyseal plate are a common musculoskeletal injury within the pediatric population with open growth plates. Such fractures represent nearly 15% to 18% of all pediatric fractures.[40–43] In 1963, Canadian orthopedic surgeons, Dr Robert B. Salter and W. Robert Harris, produced a classification system involving the physeal plate that was based on anatomy, fracture pattern, and prognosis.[43] They described two types of injuries involving the epiphyseal plate: the (1) traction epiphysis and (2) pressure epiphysis. Traction epiphyses provide appositional growth and occurs at the origin or insertion of muscles, involving the extra-articular surfaces and non-weight-bearing areas of bone.[43–45] Pressure epiphyses provide longitudinal growth and occur at the end of long bones, involving the articular surface and weight-bearing areas.[43,44] Physeal fractures consistently involve the zone of provisional calcification, which represents a transitional point between calcified and non-calcified extracellular matrix proteins, thereby making a weaker area and increasing its susceptibility to physeal injury. The ligamentous structures in children are fairly strong, whereas the physis is biomechanically vulnerable to shear and rotational forces. Therefore, the same mechanism of injury that may result in an ankle sprain in the adult population can present with a physeal or avulsion fracture in children.[34,35] Premature physeal growth arrest is one of the major complications after injury of the growth plate in children that can lead to limb deformity and limb length discrepancy.[38] The incidence of significant growth disturbance after physeal injuries in children is reported to be between 1% and 10%.[43,46]

The distal tibial physis is comprised of abundant blood supply; therefore, avascular necrosis (AVN) of the distal tibial plafond is fairly rare after a traumatic event.[47] Physeal arrest is generally not a concern after triplane ankle fractures and Tillaux fractures because of the pattern of physeal growth. The distal fibula has significant ligamentous constraint and support via the anterior tibiofibular ligament (ATFL), posterior tibiofibular ligament, and calcaneofibular ligament.[30,48] Additionally, the distal fibular physis becomes undulating during childhood, which provides it with additional stability.[30,49] Growth of the fibula is evenly distributed between the proximal and distal fibular physis in childhood, although proximal fibular growth becomes predominant in adolescents. Isolated premature physeal closure of the fibula, although rare, may result in ankle valgus and external foot progression angle.[30,50]

The most common fractures of the ankle in pediatric patients are Salter-Harris type epiphyseal fractures and avulsions from the distal aspect of the lateral malleolus. Salter Harris fractures are classified into 5 categories, which are most commonly used to describe these injuries. A Salter Harris Type I fracture is a separation through the physis; a Salter Harris Type II fracture enters in the plane of the physis and exits through the metaphysis creating a resultant Thurston-Holland fragment; a Salter Harris Type III fracture enters in the plane of the physis and exits through the epiphysis; a Salter Harris Type IV fracture transverses the physis, extending from the metaphysis to the epiphysis; and a Salter Harris Type V fracture is characterized as a crush injury of the epiphysis and physis.[19,37,43,44,51]

## TRIPLANE FRACTURE OF THE ANKLE

Triplane ankle fractures account for roughly 6% of all distal epiphyseal injuries.[52] A triplane ankle fracture most commonly occurs during adolescence at the time of partial closure of the distal tibial physis. In the triplane fracture, there is a vertical fracture of the tibial epiphysis in the sagittal plane, a horizontal fracture through the lateral part of the physis in the axial plane, and an oblique coronal fracture through the metaphysis.[53] On a frontal plain film radiograph, the fracture mimics a Salter-Harris Type III fracture of the epiphysis, whereas the lateral radiograph suggests a Salter-Harris Type II fracture.[53] The distal tibial epiphysis is the second most common site of epiphyseal fracture in the pediatric population, second to the distal radius.[54] Fractures of the tibial epiphyseal account for 5% to 10% of pediatric intra-articular ankle injuries, as boys are noted to have a higher occurrence rate than girls because of the delayed closure of the lateral tibial physis. According to Vahvanen and Aalto, their study reported an increase in predilection of left-sided ankle fractures; however, a majority of literature has noted an increase in right-sided injuries.[55] The treatment of triplane ankle fractures can be categorized into closed and open treatments.

Nondisplaced triplane ankle fractures, which are categorized as less than 2 mm of displacement and/or extra-articular fractures, can be managed with immobilization in long leg cast to prevent rotation. Closed treatment of these fractures may be performed under anesthesia and relaxation, to provide appropriate axial traction of the ankle and internal rotation of the foot.[56] Immediate plain film radiographs are necessary to obtain in the emergency department before and after reduction, in addition to postreduction CT scans, to appropriately assess the adequacy of reduction, comminution, cortical alignment, and guard against loss of reduction while the lower extremity is in a cast. Rotational malalignment, which often manifests as external rotation, will adversely affect the foot progression angle.[56,57] Triplane ankle fractures noted with greater than 2 mm of displacement will require either closed or open reduction if closed manipulation deems to be unsuccessful to restore appropriate alignment. Patients with greater than 3 mm of displacement are immediate candidates for open reduction and internal fixation because of the energy of the injury, soft-tissue and bone interposition at the fracture site, and swelling.[56,58]

Open reduction internal fixation of pediatric triplane fractures is indicated for fractures with greater than 3 mm of displacement, as well as failure to achieve adequate closed reduction, which is generally defined as greater than 2 mm of intra-articular step-off. Soft-tissue swelling and/or compromise and skin tenting must be assessed before intervention to rule out muscle and vascular compromise. The preoperative evaluation also involved multiple plain film radiographs of the foot and ankle and CT scan to aid in the treatment plan.[56] The mechanism of injury associated with triplane fracture is external rotation of the foot on the tibia, which is imperative to note as gentle internal rotation of the foot may provide appropriate alignment. The foot and ankle are then immobilized in the opposite position to the mechanism of injury.[56,59,60] Appropriate anatomic reduction, whether open or closed, is appropriate to decrease the risk of premature physeal closure, varus angulation, and shortening of the pediatric ankle.[56–62] Ertl and colleagues in 1988 published a long-term follow-up (range:

38 months to 13 years) of 23 pediatric patients who sustained a triplane ankle fractures and concluded that residual displacement greater than 2 mm was associated with poorer prognosis unless the fracture was extra-articular.[63] Barmada and colleagues in 2003 noted that residual gaps in the physis >3 mm were due to entrapped periosteum within the physis after closed reduction with splinting, which may result in an increased risk of premature physeal closure.[4] Additionally, Kling emphasized the importance of acknowledging the difficulty in performing accurate reduction of a triplane ankle fracture.[54] If the clinician is unable to attain accurate closed reduction with manipulation acutely, open management may be necessary. Kling provided a step-wise approach in addressing open management of these fractures. Open management may be achieved via Kirschner wires, partially threaded or fully threaded cannulated screws, or bioabsorbable noncannulated screw fixation to reduce internal foot print. With the patient in the supine position in the operating room, the anterolateral fragment is addressed and reduced through an anterolateral approach first. Then, the posteromedial fragment is addressed and reduced using dorsiflexion and internal rotation of the foot. Fixation should be directed from anterior to posterior direction through the anterior tibial metaphysis, to securely fix the posterior fragment and avoid the neurovascular bundle.[54] In our practice, we use absorbable 3-0 and 4-0 monocryl sutures for skin closure and place the lower extremity in a short leg cast for non-weightbearing and transition them into a controlled ankle movement boot, non-weightbearing, 7-10 days post-operative for 3-4 weeks. The patient may gradually begin physical therapy 4 to 6 weeks after the operation pending serial outpatient plain film radiographs.

## JUVENILE TILLAUX FRACTURE

Juvenile Tillaux fractures represent 2.9% of juvenile epiphyseal growth plate injuries and are characterized as an intra-articular Salter-Harris Type III fracture of the anterolateral distal tibial physis because of external rotation.[39,53,64] Tillaux fractures are fewer complex fractures than triplane ankle fractures and tend to occur later in life at the time when the anterolateral part of the distal tibial epiphysis fuses with the metaphysis.[53,65] The fracture is named after Paul Jules Tillaux, who was a French physician and the first physician to describe the Salter-Harris Type II fracture of the distal tibia.[65-70] The bony attachment of the ATFL to the epiphysis is much stronger than that of the epiphysis to the rest of the tibia; the fracture line crosses the physis and into the epiphysis. A Tillaux fracture may not be visible on a frontal radiograph because of the oblique plane of the epiphyseal fracture; therefore, the clinician should order a CT scan to confirm the presence of a Tillaux fracture.[65,71,72]

Although Tillaux fractures are rarely complicated by premature physeal closure because the majority of the epiphysis is already fused, the amount of displacement noted on imaging drives the proper treatment of a Tillaux fracture. Ideally, if displacement is less than 2 mm, the fracture may be treated nonoperatively with closed reduction, and immobilization is a long leg cast with internal rotation of the foot after ankle dorsiflexion and protonation of the foot, to prevent rotational forces.[65,72,73] Tillaux fractures with more than 2 mm of displacement and disruption of the distal tibial articular surface should be treated with open reduction and internal fixation with the use of transepiphyseal pinning or cannulated screws.[73]

## TALAR FRACTURES

Talar fractures are relatively rare injuries within the pediatric population, with an estimated prevalence of 0.008% of all childhood fractures compared with 0.3% in adults.[74] Orthopedic literature focusing on pediatric talar fracture identified motor vehicle accidents and falls from a height as the most frequent mechanisms of injury. The mechanism of injury of these fractures results from axial loading of the talus against the anterior tibia with the foot in dorsiflexion, usually due to high-energy trauma.[75–77] Older males are more commonly affected than females.[78] Jensen in 1994 and Eberl in 2010 hypothesized that this is because the pediatric foot is more flexible and skeletally immature with higher elastic resistance than adult bone; therefore, the bones are able to sustain higher forces before sustaining a fracture.[74–76] In 2010, Smith and colleagues examined 29 children with an average age of 13.5 years who sustained displaced talar fractures.[78] The study examined complications associated with these injuries and noted subtalar joint arthrosis (17%) to be the most common complication, followed by the need for further surgery (10%), AVN (7%), neuropraxia (7%), and delayed union (3%).[78] AVN of the talar body has been reported in children after minimally displaced fractures; however, AVN most likely occurs after fracture-dislocation injuries of the talus.[75–77]

Pediatric talar fractures may be classified in a similar fashion as adult talar fractures using the Hawkins classification, as majority are talar neck fractures. The original Hawkins classification included 3 fracture types: Type I through Type III. The modern version includes Type IV, which was added in 1978 by Canale and Kelly.[79,80] Hawkins Type I fractures are classified as nondisplaced or minimally displaced fractures that are verified via CT scan. Treatment for these injuries consist of closed reduction with manipulation followed by a short leg cast, or if a long leg case is placed, the knee should be flexed 30° to prevent weight-bearing. Hawkins Type II fractures are recognized as posterior displacement of the talar body and typically presents with medial comminution as the ankle joint remains congruent. Treatment consists of either closed or open reduction to appropriately reduce subtalar joint congruency with special care to avoid varus malalignment. Hawkins Type III fractures are characterized as complete posterior dislocation of the talar body with frequent internal rotation and entrapment of the posterior tibial tendon. Open reduction and internal fixation are imperative for the treatment of these injuries to restore anatomic realignment and stable osteosynthesis to prevent AVN of the talus. Postoperatively, these patients are placed into a short leg cast and allowed partial weight-bearing for 4 to 6 weeks, followed by full weight-bearing in a short leg cast for 6 to 12 weeks. Canale and Kelly added a Type IV fracture classification, which is identified by progressive impact and dislocation of the talar neck at the talonavicular joint. These fractures require open reduction internal fixation similar to those of Hawkins Type III.[10,75–83]

Meier and colleagues in 2005 examined the long-term outcome of talar neck and body fractures in 15 children with an average of 10 years (range: 4–16 years), who had been treated at an orthopedic department during a period of 21 years (range: 1976–1997) after a talar neck or body fracture.[81] They studied all Hawkins-type fractures with various treatment options. They concluded that minimally displaced (<2 mm), stable, Hawkins Type I fractures of the central talus can be treated conservatively. However, the researchers noted that other fractures of the talus should be treated surgically because there is not enough remodeling capacity at the growing skeleton and must be treated for anatomic reduction and fixation.[81]

Osteonecrosis or AVN of the talus is the most common complication associated with talar fractures in the pediatric, as well as the adult, population. This may occur due to disruption or thrombosis of the tenuous vascular supply as is associated with the initial type of injury, degree of angulation, and time to appropriate reduction. The Hawkins sign represents subchondral osteopenia in the vascularized talus approximately 6 to 8 weeks after fixation caused by resorption of the subchondral bone and is visualized as a thin subchondral radiolucent line along the talar dome on plain film radiograph.[10,82] Hawkins Type I fractures are associated with 0% to 27% incidence of talar AVN; Hawkins Type II is associated with roughly 20% to 50% risk of talar AVN. Hawkins Type III and Type IV are associated with nearly a 100% risk of talar AVN.

## CALCANEAL FRACTURES

Calcaneal fractures in skeletally immature patients are relatively uncommon and frequently missed injuries. The overall incidence of calcaneal fractures in the pediatric population has been reported to be 1 in 100,000 fractures.[84] The type of calcaneal fracture and severity typically varies with patient age, as children younger than 14 years typically have extra-articular fractures while older adolescents often sustain intra-articular injuries.[84,85] Landin, in 1983, studied 8682 fractures in children aged 16 years or less and reported the incidence of calcaneal fractures to be 0.41 per 10,000 pediatric patients.[85] Calcaneal fractures in pediatric patients are often misdiagnosed because of their subtle clinical and radiographic presentation.[86]

The primary ossification center of the calcaneus appears at 7 months in utero, the secondary ossification center appears at approximately 10 years of age, and fuses by the age of 16 years.[10] Owing to the anatomic differences between the pediatric and adult calcaneus, calcaneal fracture patterns in children differ from those of adults for three reasons: (1) Posterior facet is parallel to the ground, rather than inclined as it is in adults; (2) calcaneus is composed of an ossific nucleus surrounded by cartilage in pediatric patients, which is responsible for the dissipation of the injurious forces that produce classic fracture patterns observed in adults; and (3) the lateral process, which is responsible for calcaneal impaction, is diminutive in the immature calcaneus.[10,86–90]

Calcaneal fractures usually occur as a result of falls from a height, usually greater than 1 m.[90,91] Such a fall produces a direct shearing force creating a primary fracture and continuing axial compression with an everted foot causing a secondary impacted fracture with depression of the posterior articular facet of the calcaneus.[90–92] Although other mechanisms on injury may result in calcaneal open fractures, such as from a lawnmower incident. The Essex-Lopresti and Sanders classification are recognized as the standard classification system for calcaneal fractures; however, the Schmidt and Weiner classification system may be routinely used for pediatric calcaneal fractures.[10,93] Sanders system is the most widely used fracture classification system for calcaneal fractures. The system is based on coronal CT images and subdivides intra-articular fractures into 4 basic types depending on the number of fractures and the fracture line traversing the posterior facet of the calcaneus.[94–96]

Most orthopedic authors report that both intra-articular and extra-articular calcaneal fractures are benign entities in the pediatric population, and long-term consequences are minimum with little/no disability or dysfunction with nonoperative treatment.[86–89] Short-term outcomes after nonoperative treatment with closed reduction and immobilization have shown favorable results in short-term studies. Mora and colleagues, in 2001, looked at 22 pediatric patients with 23 fractures of the calcaneus before distal tibial physis fusion. They noted that eighteen patients (78%) of these fractures were intra-articular and five (22%) were extraarticular, and nine of the patients were followed up for 4.4 years. Of the nine fractures followed up long term, 8 were treated nonoperatively, and 1 was treated with open reduction internal fixation.[86] Seven of 9 patients were free of pain and had unrestricted foot function with no apparent gait abnormalities, and 2 of 9 patients had difficulty with activity related to climate change.[86] Consequently, the authors concluded that pediatric patients with both intraarticular and extraarticular fractures have excellent long-term prognosis.

Appropriate treatment of calcaneal fractures is highly dependent on plain film radiographs and CT imaging. Cast immobilization is recommended for pediatric patients with an extra-articular calcaneal fracture, as well as a nondisplaced or minimally displaced intra-articular fracture of the calcaneus. Weight-bearing is restricted for 6 weeks; however, children may transfer in a walking cast. Serial radiographs are warranted to monitor for joint congruency and bone remodeling to avoid severe joint depression as an indication for operative management.

Operative management of pediatric calcaneal fractures is indicated for displaced articular fractures, which typically occurs in older children and adolescents.[10,90–92] Open reduction internal fixation is warranted for displaced fractures of the anterior process of the calcaneus and severe joint depression of the middle and/or posterior facet. Anatomic reduction and restoration of the articular surface is the primary objective of surgical management of calcaneal fractures to avoid long-term complications, such as posttraumatic osteoarthritis, heel widening, varus malalignment, and nonunion.

## OTHER TARSAL FRACTURES

Fractures of the navicular, cuboid, and cuneiforms represent 5% to 7% of pediatric foot injuries.[97] Most of those injuries are avulsion or stress fractures and can usually be treated in a short walking cast for a few weeks.[98]

High-energy trauma can result in displaced fractures of the tarsal bones and can involve articulating joints. For injuries involving articular surfaces, restoration of articular surfaces is necessary which may be achieved with closed or open reduction and internal fixation.

## METATARSAL FRACTURES

Metatarsal fractures account for up to 60% of pediatric foot fractures.[99] Multiple studies reported that fifth metatarsal is the most frequently involved, while first metatarsal has the lowest incidence in children older than 5 years. In those younger than 5 years, the first metatarsal is most commonly affected.[99–101] Metatarsal injuries can occur as a result of axial loading, inversion, or rotation. It is best to assess those injuries with AP, oblique, and lateral radiographs. Lisfranc joint should be assessed. Despite the frequency of these injuries, surgical interventions are rare in closed fractures. Shaft fractures can be treated in a short leg walking cast for 3 weeks or until tenderness at the fracture site subsides. For fractures with sagittal displacement of metatarsal heads, reduction and pinning can be used to avoid transfer lesion pain.[98] In a series by Robertson and colleagues, they reported less than 3% of patients were treated surgically, Patients older than 12 years with multiple fractures and significant translation were more likely to be treated operatively. Only 4% of their cohort treated conservatively had residual pain.

Base of the 5th metatarsal fractures comprise about 40% of all metatarsal fractures and result from an inversion injury[100] and are treated based on location. Tuberosity fractures occur due to the injury at the origin of abductor digity minimi and can be treated with 6 weeks of walking cast. Those that involve the metaphyseal-diaphyseal junction or occur more distally require 6 weeks of non-weight-bearing cast. In injuries with prodromal symptoms, surgical treatment may be considered.[98] Patients older than 13 years and those with preceding stress injury at this site are at the highest risk of nonunion.[102]

## PHALANGEAL FRACTURES

Although very common in the pediatric population, those injuries are often treated at home. Closed fractures rarely require intervention and can be treated with buddy taping and/or a hard-sole shoe. Angulated or intraarticular fractures may be treated with reduction and pinning. Operative treatment is recommended for intraarticular fractures of the proximal phalanx of the hallux if more than 30% of the articular surface is involved or there is more than 3 mm of displacement.[102] Close attention should be paid to the skin and nail bed of the distal phalanx fractures because this fracture pattern can often result in osteomyelitis when not treated in time. Treatment with irrigation and debridement, stabilization, and antibiotic administration is warranted.[103]

## DISCLOSURE

The authors have nothing to disclose.

## REFERENCES

1. Danesco ER, Miller TR, Spicer RS. Incidence and costs of 1987-1994 childhood injuries: demographic breakdowns. Pediatrics 2000;105(2):e27.
2. O'Dell MC, Jaramillo D, Bancroft L, et al. Imaging of sports-related injuries of the lower extremity in pediatric patients. Radiographics 2016;36(6):1807–27.
3. Olgun ZD, Maestre S. Management of pediatric ankle fractures. Curr Rev Musculoskelet Med 2018;11:475–84.
4. Barmada A, Gaynor T, Mubarak SJ. Premature physeal closure following distal tibia physeal fractures: a new radiographic predictor. J Pediatr Orthop 2003;23:733–9.
5. Maffulli N, Giai Via A, Oliva F. Acute lower extremity injuries in pediatric and adolescent sports. In: Caine D, Purcell L, editors. Injury in pediatric and adolescent sports. contemporary pediatric and adolescent sports medicine. Cham: Springer; 2016.
6. Bruns W, Maffulli N. Lower limb injuries in children in sports. Clin Sports Med 2000;19:637–62.
7. Wuerz TH, Gurd DP. Pediatric physeal ankle fracture. J Am Acad Orthop Surg 2013;21(4):234–44.
8. Vitale M. Epidemiology of fractures in children. In: Beaty JH, Kasser JR, editors. Rockwood and Wilkins fractures in children. 7th edition. Philadelphia: Lippincott Williams and Wilkins; 2010.
9. Wimberly Robert L. General principles of managing orthopaedic injuries. Tachdjian's pediatric orthopedics. 5th edition. Saunders; 2014.
10. Egol KA, Kovak KJ, Zuckerman JD. Pediatric orthopedic surgery (Chp. 42): general principles. Handbook of fractures. 6th edition 2020.
11. Hamilton BE, Hoyert DL, Martin JA, et al. Annual summary of vital statistics: 2010-2011. Pediatrics 2013;131(3):548–58.
12. Arias E, MacDorman MF, Strobino DM, et al. Annual summary of vital statistics. Pediatrics 2003;112(6 Pt 1):1215–30.
13. Densmore JC, Lim HJ, Oldham KT, et al. Outcomes and delivery of care in pediatric injury. J Pediatr Surg 2006;41(1):92–8.
14. Stylianos S, Egorova N, Guice KS, et al. Variation in treatment of pediatric spleen injury at trauma centers verses nontrauma centers: a call for dissemination of American Pediatric Surgical Association benchmarks guidelines. J AM Coll Surg 2006;202(2):247–51.

15. Kingsnorth J, O'Connell K, Guzzetta CE, et al. Family presence during trauma activations and medical resuscitations in a pediatric emergency department: an evidence-based practice project. J Emerg Nurs 2010;36(2):115–21.
16. Carty H. Accessory ossicles at the lateral malleolus: a review of the incidence. Eur J Radiol 1992;14:181–4.
17. Stiell IG, Greenberg GH, McKnight RD, et al. A study to develop clinical decision rules for the use of radiography in acute ankle injuries. Ann Emerg Med 1992;21(4):384–90.
18. Seifert J, Matthes G, Hinz P, et al. Role of magnetic resonance imaging in the diagnosis of distal tibia fractures in adolescents. J Pediatr Orthop 2003;23(6):727–32.
19. Tachj.
20. Davis KW. Imaging pediatric sports injuries: lower extremity. Radiol Clin North Am 2010 Nov;48(6):1213–35.
21. Lawson JP, Keller MS, Rattner Z. Recent advances in pediatric musculoskeletal imaging. Radiol Clin North Am 1994;32:353–75.
22. Jaramillo D, Hoffer FA. Cartilaginous epiphysis and growth plate: normal and abnormal MR imaging findings. AJR Am J Roentgenol 1992;158:1105–10.
23. Jaramillo D, Hoffer FA, Shapiro F, et al. MR imaging of fracture of the growth plate. AJR 1990;155:1261–5.
24. Jaramillo D, Shapiro F, Hoffer FA, et al. Post-traumatic growth-plate abnormalities: MR imaging of bony bridge formation in rabbits. Radiology 1990;175:767–73.
25. Kern M, Tucker A, Rogers K, et al. CT utilization for pediatric orthopedic trauma. Del Med J 2015;87(12):366–9.
26. Wehner T, Claes L, Simon U. Internal loads in the human tibia during gait. Clin Biomech 2009;24(3):299–302.
27. Hof AL, Geelen BA, Van den Berg J. Calf muscle moment, work and efficiency in level walking; role of series elasticity. J Biomech 1983;16:523–37.
28. Su AW, Larson AN. Pediatric ankle fractures: concepts and treatment principles. Foot Ankle Clin 2015;20(4):705–19.
29. Gogi N, Deriu L. Common paediatric lower limb injuries. Surgery (Oxford) 2017;35(1):27–32.
30. Rhinelander FW. Blood supply to developing mature and healing bone. Philadelphia (PA): WB Saunders; 1982. p. 81.
31. Rhinelander FW. Tibial blood supply in relation to fracture healing. Clin Orthop Relat Res 1974;105:34–81.
32. Crock HV. The blood supply of the lower limb bones in man. Edinburg & London: E. & S. Livingston Ltd.; 1967.
33. Strachan RK, McCarthy I, Fleming R, et al. The role of the tibial nutrient artery. Microsphere estimation of blood flow in the osteotomised canine tibia. J Bone Joint Surg Br 1990;72:391–4.
34. Dingeman RD, Shaver GD. Operative treatment of displaced Salter-Harris III distal tibial fractures. Clin Orthop Rel Res 1978;135:101–3.
35. Rogers LF. The radiography of epiphyseal injuries. Radiology 1970;96:289–99.
36. Langenskiold A. Traumatic premature closure of the distal tibial epiphyseal plate. Acta Orthop Scand 1967;38:520–31.
37. Salter RB. Injuries of the ankle in children. Orthop Clin North Am 1974;5:147–52.
38. Hajdu S, Schwendenwein E, Kaltenecker G, et al. Growth potential of different zones of the growth plate-an experimental study in rabbits. J Orthop Res 2012;30:162–8.

39. Chaudhry S, Dehne K. Ankle fractures in children. Open J Trauma 2019;3(1): 018–21.
40. Mizuta T, Benson WM, Foster BK, et al. Statistical analysis of the incidence of physeal injuries. J Pediatr Orthop 1987;7:518–23.
41. Rogers LF. The radiography of epiphyseal injuries. Radiology 1970;96: 289–99. 25.
42. Rohmiller MT, Gaynor TP, Pawelek J, et al. Salter-Harris I and II fractures of the distal tibia: does mechanism of injury relate to premature physeal closure? J Pediatr Orthop 2006;26:322–8. 26.
43. Salter RB, Harris WR. Injuries involving the epiphyseal plate. J Bone Joint Surg Am 1963;45:587–622.
44. Cepela DJ, Tartaglione JP, Dooley TP, et al. Classifications in brief: Salter-Harris classification of pediatric physeal fractures. Clin Orthop Relat Res 2016;474(11): 2531–7.
45. Reginelli A, Russo A, Turrizziani F, et al. Imaging of pediatric foot disorders. Acta Biomed 2018;89(1-S):34–47.
46. Mizuta T, Benson WM, Foster BK, et al. Statistical analysis of the incidence of physeal injuries. J Pediatr Orthop 1987;7:518–23.
47. Su AW, Larson AN. Pediatric ankle fractures. Foot Ankle Clin 2015;20(4):705–19.
48. Hertel J. Functional anatomy, pathomechanics, and pathophysiology of lateral ankle instability. J Athl Train 2002;37(4):364–75.
49. Ogden JA, McCarthy SM. Radiology of postnatal skeletal development. VIII. Distal tibia and fibula. Skeletal Radiol 1983;10:209–20.
50. Pritchett JW. Growth and growth prediction of the fibula. Clin Orthop Relat Res 1997;(334):251–6.
51. Stephens DC, Louis E, Louis DS. Traumatic separation of the distal femoral epiphyseal cartilage plate. J Bone Joint Surg Am 1974;56(7):1383–90.
52. Ramsden W. Fractures and musculoskeletal trauma. In: Carty H, editor. Emergency pediatric radiology. Berlin: Springer-Verlag; 1999. p. 313–34.
53. Vanhoenacker FM, Bernaerts A, Gielen J, et al. Trauma of the pediatric ankle and foot. JBR-BTR 2002;85(4):212–8.
54. Kling TF Jr. Operative treatment of ankle fractures in children. Orthop Clin North Am 1990;21:381–92.
55. Vahvanen V, Aalto K. Classification of ankle fractures in children. Arch Orthop Trauma Surg 1980;97:1–5.
56. Schnetzler KA, Hoernschemeyer D. The pediatric triplane ankle fracture. J Am Acad Orthop Surg 2007;15(12):738–47.
57. Phan VC, Wroten E, Yngve DA. Foot progression angle after distal tibial physeal fractures. J Pediatr Orthop 2002;22:31–5.
58. Kay RM, Matthys GA. Pediatric ankle fractures: evaluation and treatment. J Am Acad Orthop Surg 2001;9:268–78.
59. Dias LS, Giegerich CR. Fractures of the distal tibial epiphysis in adolescence. J Bone Joint Surg Am 1983;65:438–44.
60. Dias LS, Tachdjian MO. Physeal injuries of the ankle in children: classification. Clin Orthop Relat Res 1978;136:230–3.
61. Kärrholm J. The triplane fracture: Four years of follow-up of 21 cases and review of the literature. J Pediatr Orthop B 1997;6:91–102.
62. Kling TF Jr, Bright RW, Hensinger RN. Distal tibial physeal fractures in children that may require open reduction. J Bone Joint Surg Am 1984;66:647–57.
63. Ertl JP, Barrack RL, Alexander AH, et al. Triplane fracture of the distal tibial epiphysis: long-term follow-up. J Bone Joint Surg Am 1988;70:967–76.

64. Spiegel PG, Cooperman DR, Laros GS. Epiphyseal fractures of the distal ends of the tibia and fibula. A retrospective study of two hundred and thirty-seven cases in children. J Bone Joint Surg Am 1978;60(8):1046–50.

65. Habusta SF, Ponnarasu S, Mabrouk A, et al. Tillaux fracture. 2021.

66. Haller JM, Githens M, Rothberg D, et al. Risk factures for tibial plafond nonunion: medial column fixation may reduce nonunion rates. J Orthop Trauma 2019;33(9):443–9.

67. Mathieu L, Mongo V, Potier L, et al. Type III open tibia fractures in low-resources setting. Part 3: achievement of bone union and treatment of segmental bone defects. Med Sante Trop 2019;29(1):36–42.

68. Tuca M, Bernal N, Luderowski E, et al. Tibial spine avulsion fractures: treatment update. Curr Opin Pediatr 2019;31(1):103–11.

69. Pires J, Oliveira S, Figueiredo P, et al. Rehabilitation of simultaneous bilateral epiphysial fracture of proximal tibia in adolescent. BMJ Case Rep 2018.

70. Mijatović D, Orehovec SS, Đapić T, et al. Management of a complex lower limb open fracture in a teenage patient: a case report. Ostomy Wound Manag 2018; 64(5):47–52.

71. Schlesinger I, Wedge JH. Percutaneous reduction and fixation of displaced juvenile Tillaux fractures: a new surgical technique. J Pediatr Orthop 1993;13(3): 389–91.

72. Choudhry IK, Wall EJ, Eismann EA, et al. Functional outcome analysis of triplane and tillaux fractures after closed reduction and percutaneous fixation. J Pediatr Orthop 2014;34(2):139–43.

73. Kaya A, Altay T, Ozturk H, et al. Open reduction and internal fixation in displaced juvenile Tillaux fractures. Injury 2007;38(2):201–5.

74. Thermann H, Schratt HE, Hufner T, et al. Fractures of the pediatric foot. Unfallchirurgie 1998;101:2–11.

75. Jensen I, JU Wester, Rasmussen F, et al. Prognosis of fracture of the talus in children. 21 (7-34)-year follow-up of 14 cases. Acta Orthop Scand 1994;65: 398–400.

76. Eberl R, Singer G, Schalamon J, et al. Fractures of the talus–differences between children and adolescents. J Trauma 2010;68:126–30.

77. Cartwright-Terry M, Pullen H. Non-operative management of a talar body fracture in a skeletally immature patient. Acta Orthop Belg 2008;74:137–40.

78. Smith JT, Curtis TA, Spencer S, et al. Complications of talus fractures in children. J Pediatr Orthop 2010;30:779–84.

79. Alton T, Patton DJ, Gee AO. Classifications in brief: the hawkins classification for talus fractures. Clin Orthop Relat Res 2015;473:3046–9.

80. Canale ST, Kelly FB Jr. Fractures of the neck of the talus: long-term evaluation of seventy-one cases. J Bone Joint Surg Am 1978;60:143–56.

81. Meier R, Krettek C, Griensven M, et al. Fractures of the talus in the pediatric patient. J Foot Ankle 2005;11(1):5–10.

82. DeValentine S, Blakeslee T, Schuberth J. Fractures in children. In: Scurran BL, editor. Foot and ankle trauma. St Louis: Churchill Livingstone; 1995. p. 257–362.

83. Pearce DH, Mongiardi CN, Fornasier VL, et al. Avascular necrosis of the talus: a pictorial essay. RadioGraphics 2005;25(2):399–410.

84. Wiley JJ, Profitt A. Fractures of the os calcis in children. Clin Orthop Relat Res 1984;(188):131–8.

85. Schantz K, Rasmussen F. Calcaneus fracture in the child. Acta Orthop Scand 1987;58(5):507–9.

86. Mora S, Thordarson DB, Zionts LE, et al. Pediatric calcaneal fractures. Foot Ankle Int 2001;22(6):471–7.
87. Chapman HG, Galway HR. Os calcis fractures in childhood. J Bone Joint Surg 1977;58B:510.
88. DeBeer JDV, Maloon 5, Hudson DA. Calcaneal fractures in children. S Afr Med J 1989;76:53–4.
89. Jonasch E. Fersenbeinbruche bei kindern. Hefte Unfallheilkd 1979;134:170.
90. Najefi A-A, Najefy A, Vemulapalli K. Paediatric calcaneal fractures: a guide to management based on a review of the literature. Injury 2020.
91. Schantz K, Rasmussen F. Calcaneus fracture in the child. Acta Orthop Scand 1987;58(5):507–9.
92. Thomas HM. Calcaneal fracture in childhood. Br J Surg 1969;56(9):664–6.
93. Schmidt TL, Weiner DS. Calcaneal fractures in children. An evaluation of the nature of the injury in 56 children. Clin Orthop Relat Res 1982;171:150–5.
94. Sanders R, Fortin P, DiPasquale T, et al. Operative treatment in 120 displaced intraarticular calcaneal fractures. Results using a prognostic computed tomography scan classification. Clin Orthop Relat Res 1993;290:87–95.
95. Masciocchi C, Conchiglia A, Conti L, et al. Imaging of insufficiency fractures. Geriatric Imaging: Springer-Verlag Berlin Heidelberg; 2013. p. 83–91.
96. Galluzzo M, Greco F, Pietragalla M, et al. Calcaneal fractures: radiological and CT evaluation and classification systems. Acta Biomed 2018;89(1-S):138–50.
97. Crawford AH. Fractures and dislocations of the foot and ankle, skeletal trauma in children. Philadelphia: WB Sauners; 1994. p. 449–516.
98. Kay RM, Tang CW. Pediatric foot fractures: evaluation and treatment. J Am Acad Orthop Surg 2001;9:308–19.
99. Robertson N, Roocroft J, Edmonds E. Childhood metatarsal shaft fractures: treatment outcomes and relative indications for surgical intervention. J Child Orthop 2012;6:125–9.
100. Owen RJ, Hickey FG, Finlay DB. A study of metatarsal fractures in children. Injury 1995;26(8):537–8.
101. Singer G, Cichocki M, Schalamon J, et al. A study of metatarsal fractures in children. J Bone Joint Surg Am 2008;90(4):772–6.
102. Denning J. Complications of pediatric foot and ankle fractures. Orthop Clin North Am 2017;48:59–70.
103. Baker CE, Leafblad N, Larson AN. Pediatric seymour fractures of the toe. J Pediatr Orthop 2021;41(1):e55–9.

# Pediatric Forefoot Deformities

Maryellen P. Brucato, DPM[a],*, David Y. Lin, MD[b]

## KEYWORDS

- Polydactyly • Syndactyly • Macrodactyly • Congenital hallux varus • Curly toe
- Underlapping fifth toe

## KEY POINTS

- Congenital forefoot deformities can be genetically complex because of multiple signaling pathways and genes involved with limb formation.
- Polydactyly surgical correction is not a simple amputation of the extranumerary toe(s) and can require complex surgical planning and reconstruction.
- Syndactyly should not always be treated with surgical intervention, especially when only for the purposes of cosmesis.
- Underlapping curly toes often fail conservative treatment and if they do not spontaneously resolve, surgical tenotomies have good outcomes.
- Congenital hallux varus is often associated with polydactyly and surgical correction should be focused on soft tissue balancing.
- Surgical correction of macrodactyly is the mainstay for treatment and requires long-term follow-up due to likelihood of recurring complications.

## INTRODUCTION

The development of the lower extremity starts with limb bud formation between the fourth and eighth weeks of gestation.[1] The limb buds arise from the trunk and form along 3 asymmetrical axes with the lower limb lagging behind the upper extremity for a few days.[1,2] Toes differentiate typically in the seventh week.[3] There are 2 different signaling centers: the apical ectodermal ridge and the zone of polarizing activity.[1] Limb development is linked to multiple genes and encoding proteins.[1] Thus, congenital forefoot deformities can be genetically intricate with high phenotypic variability.

## DEFINITIONS, EPIDEMIOLOGY, AND CLASSIFICATIONS OF POLYDACTYLY

Polydactyly is a congenital limb malformation that results in the presence of supernumerary digit(s) and/or metatarsals.[4,5] It may present as a complete duplication of a

[a] Brucato Foot and Ankle Surgery, LLC, 1011 Clifton Avenue, Suite 1G, Clifton, NJ 07013, USA;
[b] The Pediatric Orthopedic Center, 218 Ridgedale Avenue, Suite 101, Cedar Knolls, NJ 07927, USA
* Corresponding author.
E-mail address: brucatofootsx@gmail.com

Clin Podiatr Med Surg 39 (2022) 73–87
https://doi.org/10.1016/j.cpm.2021.08.002
0891-8422/22/© 2021 Elsevier Inc. All rights reserved.
podiatric.theclinics.com

digit including all soft tissue and osseous structures.[5] Although it is phenotypically variable, it is highly heterogeneous.[6]

The epidemiology of polydactyly is scant because it is not registered as a congenital anomaly. From a 1960 study, the incidence has been most commonly reported as approximately 1.7 per 1000 live births.[7] A newer study performed in the Netherlands in 2013 reported an incidence of 8.4 patients per 10,000 live births[8] and a study from 2014 estimated incidence to be 0.3 to 3.6 per 1000 live births.[6]

Polydactyly can be an isolated deformity, part of a congenital syndrome, and/or associated with other anatomic anomalies.[2] It is most often associated with hand polydactyly as well as syndactyly.[2,9] Some syndromes it is commonly associated with include: Ellis Van Creveld syndrome, trisomy 13, tibial hemimelia, trisomy 21, and Greig cephalopolysyndactyly.[9] Sporadic cases are usually unilateral, whereas familial cases tend to be bilateral and symmetric.[6] Approximately, 30% of cases have a positive family history.[2,10] Typically, polydactyly is autosomal-dominant inheritance with variable penetrance.[11] However, it is not always a Mendelian inheritance because it is polygenic involves several signaling factors primarily the sonic hedgehog (SHH) genes and the HOX genes. The Gli3 gene has been identified as one focus in particular.[4,9]

Temtamy and McKusick separated polydactyly into 3 main groups based on the location of the deformity only: preaxial, postaxial, and central ray.[5] The preaxial and postaxial duplications have different patterns of genetic inheritance.[9]

- Preaxial (medial) 15% of cases
- Postaxial (lateral) 80% of cases
  - Type A fully developed digit with duplication of all structures
  - Type B soft tissue duplication
  - Type M combination of A & B
- Central ray duplication (2, 3, or 4) 5% of cases.[2]

In addition, Venn Watson created a polydactyly classification based on the shape of the associated metatarsal bone (**Fig. 1**). This represents a simple classification of 6 different types and therefore not all cases can be classified by Venn Watson.[12] Others have published their own distinct classification systems including the SAM classification that was created for surgical planning as well as Watanabe.[13]

## SYMPTOMS

Although this deformity is present at birth, parents may be hesitant to seek surgical evaluation while the child is young. It is typical in our practice to have older children in the 8 to 12 years old range present for treatment for the first time. Complaints include difficulty fitting in shoes, pain from supernumerary digit rubbing on shoes, deformity, and unfavorable cosmesis. Preaxial polydactyly is also associated with hallux varus.[11]

## IMAGING

Radiographic evaluation is essential for surgical planning. Dorsoplantar and lateral views are the most appropriate to assess the deformity. In addition, an MRI may be desirable when choosing which digit to excise as it can demonstrate what structures exist for each toe. Particularly helpful is the evaluation of the extensor and flexor tendon insertions, which is not always evident by physical examination.[2]

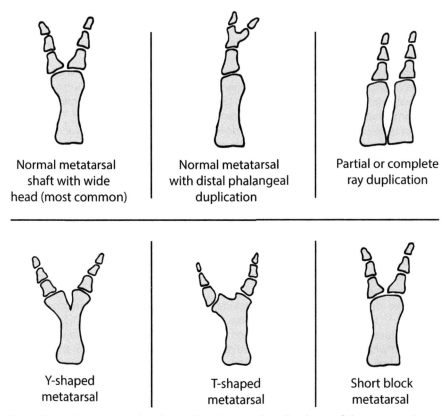

| Normal metatarsal shaft with wide head (most common) | Normal metatarsal with distal phalangeal duplication | Partial or complete ray duplication |
| Y-shaped metatarsal | T-shaped metatarsal | Short block metatarsal |

**Fig. 1.** Venn Watson's polydactyly classification based on the shape of the associated metatarsal bone.

## SURGICAL MANAGEMENT

What is the optimal age for polydactyly correction? This question remains somewhat controversial. Straightforward deformities that can be treated by simple amputation can be performed as soon as the patient is able to tolerate anesthesia safely.[2] For more complex deformities that require osteotomies or some type of reconstruction, we recommend waiting until the patient is at least 1 year old.[2] Of course, this should be considered on a case-by-case basis. A study published in 2007 reported an average of corrections at 3.9 years old.[14] A 2018 study by Kubat and colleagues reported no significant difference in final outcome between early and late interventions in 24 consecutive patients in 2 groups "early" with a median age of 1 year old and "late" with a median age of 8.5 years old.[15]

Surgical goals include:

- More narrow foot to fit in shoes
- Stabilized foot
- Well balanced foot
- Normal foot contour
- Maintain joint stability with soft tissue balancing
- Improved cosmesis[2]

The selection of which digit to remove should be assessed on a case-by-case basis. If the remaining toes are all within normal limits, it is recommended to remove either the most medial or the most lateral supernumerary digit.[10] All duplicated bones should be excised.[2]

For preaxial cases, you would not excise the most medial if it is more developed than the duplicated digit. This would require a reattachment of the adductor hallucis to prevent hallux varus.[2] Preaxial surgical technique often involves correcting a hallux varus component. These are known to have poorer surgical outcomes.[12] There are a variety of techniques described to close down first ray splaying and prevent widening of the overtime including plication of adductor hallucis and resection of excess skin and subcutaneous tissue in the first webspace.[12]

In postaxial cases, sometimes the fifth toe is smaller than the sixth toe and thus the smaller toe should be excised.[2] If both fifth and sixth toes are short, Togashi described a surgical technique using an island flap from the extranumerary toe to lengthen the remaining toe.[16]

Surgical correction for central ray polydactyly tends to be more complex. Even after excision, it is difficult to create a narrow foot.[14] Various incision techniques can be used including racquet type and wedge resection with dorsal and plantar incisions. Even when there is not a tarsal duplication cuneiform excision may be required to create a narrow foot.[2]

If angular deformities exist in the metatarsals, they may require osteotomies for correction.[14] It is critical to maintain the extensor and flexor attachments to the remaining toes with meticulous dissection.[2] In cases where there is a widened metatarsal head with 2 toes, disarticulate and detach collateral ligament from the excised toe and suture it back to the remaining toe for stabilization.[2] A Kirschner wire can always be used to maintain stability and removed in office in 4 to 6 weeks.[2,11] In addition, reconstruction of the intermetatarsal ligament should be performed if indicated to help bring metatarsals together.[2] Reapproximation of the metatarsals could also be performed by suturing or cerclaging them together.[2]

Whenever performing these procedures, it is recommended to take the tourniquet down before closing or consider doing the procedure wet.[2]

## SURGICAL COMPLICATIONS

Hallux varus is a common complication of preaxial polydactyly correction. This is usually treated with syndactylization of the first and second toes.[11] Because of rebalancing of the foot, transfer metatarsalgias can occur.[11] Widening of the foot over time can also occur because of destabilization.[2]

## SUMMARY

Surgery is not always straightforward, requires careful planning on a case-by-case basis. It requires flexibility and personalization of surgical techniques but can be very successful. Turra and colleagues reported surgical results on 42 patients with 55 duplications. Sixty-six percent had excellent results, 25% had good results, and 9% had poor results. Four of 5 of the poor results were preaxial polydactyly and had problems with hallux varus or incomplete bony resection.

## CLINIC CARE POINTS

- Polydactyly can be an isolated deformity, part of a congenital syndrome, or associated with other anomalies

- Genetic inheritance patterns vary greatly and are not yet completely understood
- The deformity needs to be fully evaluated and preoperative planning needs to be individualized for each child
- Surgical planning may not be as easy as simply amputating the extra digit
- Consider reconstructing collateral ligaments, tendons, and deep intermetatarsal ligament to prevent hallux varus or widening of the foot over time

## DEFINITIONS, EPIDEMIOLOGY, AND CLASSIFICATIONS OF SYNDACTYLY

Syndactyly is another congenital limb malformation that occurs when toes fail to separate during organogenesis. This results in webbing between toes.[6] The incidence ranges from 1 in 2000 to 1 in 2500.[17] It can be syndromic or nonsyndromic[4] (**Fig. 2**).

Although it is considered an inherited deformity, there have been cases documented that did not have any familial history.[1,4] It usually follows autosomal dominant inheritance; however, 2 autosomal recessive types have been identified. In addition, an X-linked recessive type has been identified. The Mendelian dominant type is usually less severe with wide variability of expression with incomplete penetrance. This can result in interfamilial and intrafamilial phenotypic variabilities.[6]

There is a wide variety of presentations with interlimb phenotypic variation:

- Mild, moderate, or severe webbing
- Unilateral or bilateral
- Symmetric or asymmetrical
- Complete or incomplete
- Cutaneous or bony[4,6]

The most widely used syndactyly classification system is Temtamy and McKusick. It is based on the phenotype and pattern of disease in large families and also includes the hands. It identifies 5 discrete syndactylies; however, typing can be difficult because of overlapping phenotypes. Furthermore, classification of syndactyly is not critical.[6]

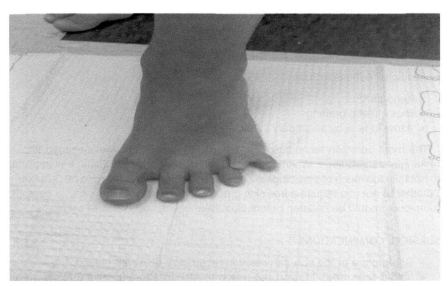

**Fig. 2.** Polydactyly shown with an extra 5th digit is another congenital limb malformation that occurs when toes fail to separate during organogenesis.

## IS SURGICAL INTERVENTION REQUIRED?

This remains a somewhat controversial subject. Tachdijan stated that syndactyly is cosmetic only and does not require surgical treatment. However, one must consider the psychological impact of the deformity on a child.[17] Moreover, surgery is requested commonly for children in Asian countries and communities due to customs involving the removal of shoes in the house.[18]

What is the optimal age for surgery? This has not been studied in detail but Langlais and colleagues published a study that showed patients who underwent desyndactylization before the age of 2 years had higher rates of long-term satisfaction and lower rates of recurrence. However, they noted this could lead to more bone deformations due to higher growth potential.

## SURGICAL TECHNIQUE

Surgical techniques can be divided into 2 different categories: open versus closed. When performing a desyndactylization, a skin defect is created as the surface area of the toes increases. An open technique creates a skin defect large enough to require skin grafting, whereas a closed technique uses flaps to cover the entire defect.

Countless types of flaps including shapes and configurations have been published:

- V shape[5]
- Z shape[5]
- Rectangular shape[5]
- Three square flap[19]
- Pentagonal island flap[20]
- Interdigitating triangular flaps[21]
- Straight linear incision with elliptical-shaped flap[22]

For open techniques, authors have described several different donor sites for free skin grafts:

- Pinch graft from lateral calcaneus[5]
- Pinch graft from medial ankle[22]
- Skin graft from polydactyly resection if concomitant deformity exists[5]
- Rectangle shaped from arch of foot[21]

Additional options include:

- Xenograft[5]
- Biosynthetic grafting
- Allow to heal by secondary intent[17]

The most common techniques that we use in our practice are V-shaped flaps or rectangle-shaped flaps. When performing the dissection of the flaps, it is important to not take too much of the adipose tissue layer. This layer may need to be debulked.[22] Whether or not you require a free skin graft and what size will vary case to case. The tourniquet should be deflated before closure to check vascularity of skin flaps.

## SURGICAL COMPLICATIONS

- Contracture of the scar can result in recurrence AKA web creep[5,21]
- Keloid scar. Keep in mind patients with African ethnicity have a higher rate of keloid formation[17]
- Frontal and/or sagittal plane[17,18]

- Donor site morbidity from free flaps
- Postoperative defects from failed flaps on surgical site[5]
- Neurovascular compromise[5]

Marsh and colleagues performed a study on 15 consecutive patients with 19 toes treated with triangular-shaped flaps and split thickness skin graft from the arch. Only one patient had recurrence.[21] Another study in 2017 described 66 cases that were treated with a linear incision dorsally and the skin defect was covered with pinch graft from the ankle.[22]

## SUMMARY

The decision for surgical management should be carefully weighed for each patient because it is typically not fixing a functional problem. We highly recommend against operating for cosmesis, especially because postoperative cosmesis may not be ideal. Scarring and asymmetry are common complications. Complication rates can be as high as 11.7%.[17] Recurrence can be as high as 28%.[17] It is important to discuss all the potential complications with the parents including disappointing cosmetic results.[17]

## CLINIC CARE POINTS

- Carefully consider operative treatment on a case-by-case basis because of unfavorable cosmetic results and potentially high recurrence and complication rates.
- Two distinct surgical techniques are described: open (requiring a skin graft) and closed (not requiring a skin graft)
- No studies have shown a significant advantage over flap shapes or surgical techniques

## CURLY TOES (UNDERLAPPING TOES)
### Introduction/History/Definitions/Background

Congenital curly toes are relatively common, generally asymptomatic, soft tissue deformities of the lesser lateral toes of which the third and fourth toes are most commonly affected.[23,24] Children are often brought into pediatricians' offices for evaluation because of familial concerns. It has been estimated to affect about 2.8% to 3% of the population.[25] Owing to flexor tendon (flexor digitorum brevis [FDB] and flexor digitorum longus [FDL]) intrinsic tightness or congenital shortening, and flexor/extensor tendon imbalance, the affected toe is flexed, adducted, and laterally rotated at the proximal and/or distal interphalangeal joint levels. The adjacent and medial overriding toe is often mistaken as the digit with the pathology when it is the lateral underlapping toe pushing it upwards. Curly toes are often bilateral, although unilateral cases are not infrequent, and have no known cause or genetic predisposition[23-26] (Fig. 3).

The overpowering pull of these plantar tendons causes the affected digit to underlap the neighboring medial digit in varying severities. The vast majority of these deformities are supple and easily and passively correctable, with rare instances of true contractures. In 25% to 50% of cases, curly toes resolve spontaneously especially in early childhood so initial observation, watchful waiting, and parental reassurance is warranted even up to age 6 years.[23,27] Stretching, strapping, or taping techniques for curly toes have been shown to be ineffective in previous studies.[24,25]

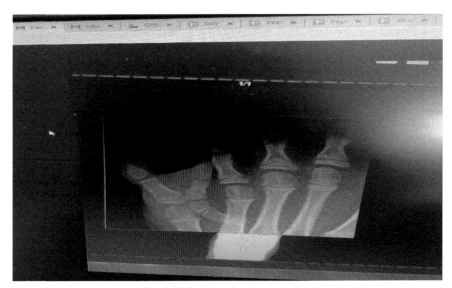

**Fig. 3.** An AP X-ray image of the Clinical picture shown in **Fig. 2.**

Surgical correction is indicated if the child develops shoe wear issues, gait disturbances, functional limitations, contractures, or signs of skin irritation (eg, calluses,
blisters, nail changes, toe pain, hyperkeratosis, abrasions). A softer indication for surgical intervention is for cosmetic reasons, especially in female patients.[24]

Surgical procedures to correct curly toes range from simple open flexor tenotomies
(FDL ± FDB)[24,28–31] to more involved flexor-to-extensor tendon transfers (Girdle-
stone).[32] Although results have been similar for both,[9] the technique for open tenotomies is preferred because of its low learning curve, ease of execution, favorable
results, and lower complication rates.[28,30]

### Author's Preferred Surgical Technique

With the child supine and under anesthesia, a calf or ankle tourniquet is applied and
inflated. With the surgeon sitting at the end of the operating table, a longitudinal or
oblique incision is made through the skin along the plantar surface of the proximal
phalanx. If a longitudinal incision is made, be wary of crossing the flexor creases to
reduce chances of postoperative soft tissue contractures. Hemostasis is achieved
with electrocautery. Blunt and sharp dissection is carried down toward the flexor
sheath. Be wary of the neuromuscular bundles along the medial and lateral edges
of the incision. The sheath is divided lengthwise to expose the tendons. Using a small
hemostat, the FDB and FDL tendons are delivered out of the incision and are transected sharply. The skin incision is closed with absorbable sutures. Local anesthetic
is administered as a digital block. A sterile dressing is applied to keep the digit straight
and in a corrected position. The patient is permitted to weight bear with a hard sole
shoe and follow-up is approximately 7 to 10 days postoperative.

### Clinic Care Points

- Curly toes are soft tissue, flexion deformities of the lateral lesser toes causing the
  digit to underlap the adjacent medial toe due to tight flexor tendons.

- Conservative management including taping, strapping and stretching is ineffective, although spontaneous correction may occur in some younger children.
- Surgical open tenotomies of the FDB and FDL of the affected toe are very effective and successful in correcting the deformity.

## CONGENITAL HALLUX VARUS

Congenital hallux varus (CHV) is a rare condition presenting at birth involving medial angulation of the great toe at the level of the first metatarsal phalangeal joint. It is also known as an atavistic great toe. There are varying degrees of angular deviation from a few degrees to up to 90°. The condition can present in isolation or combined with other malformations such as polydactyly, metatarsus primus varus, skeletal dysplasia, or clubfoot. Typically, it is a product of an imbalance between the great toe abductors and adductors. It is frequently associated with a cordlike thickened band of the abductor hallucis along the medial MTP joint, short and broad first metatarsal, and the presence of a longitudinal epiphyseal first metatarsal bracket (LEB).[33,34] In addition, supernumerary bones or polydactyly of the phalanges and metatarsals simultaneously and frequently occur within the same foot. There is no genetic predilection for this condition.[35–40]

Besides an obvious cosmetic deformity and broadening of the forefoot, CHV poses difficulty with shoe wear, causes soft tissue irritation, and affects weight-bearing activities of daily life. Diagnosis of hallux varus is made upon clinical evaluation and foot radiographs (weight-bearing AP, lateral and oblique views).[33] Computed tomography (CT) scanning may be helpful for preoperative planning, which usually requires a combination of bony and soft tissue procedures to correct bony deformities and to balance muscle and ligamentous forces. MRI of the foot can better delineate epiphyseal bars. Goals of treatment are to provide a plantigrade, stable, and pain-free foot that can fit shoes without recurrence.

Because of its varying presentations, surgical management is tailored to the soft tissue and bony pathology presented. Typically, lengthening of tissues alongside the medial forefoot is required as the hallux is realigned causing a soft tissue deficit. When indicated, an osteotomy may be performed.[35] Soft tissue coverage of this side of the foot is supplied usually by a proximally base rotational flap taken from excess tissue found either dorsally or along the plantar surface along the widened first webspace. Surgical release of the longitudinal bracket, if present, is required to reduce chances of recurrence. The abductor hallucis is lengthened. Supernumerary bones are removed as needed.[35–37]

In 1958, Farmer[36] reported on 8 cases presenting at Hospital for Sick Children in Toronto over an 11-year span emphasizing its rarity. Similar to most of the cases was a medial transverse incision placed at the first MTP joint to release and lengthen the soft tissues followed by the previously described rotational flap.

McElvenny[33] described 4 anatomic characteristics of CHV that included: (1) shortened first metatarsal; (2) accessory bones/toes; (3) varus deformity of one or more metatarsals, and (4) a firm fibrous band/tether that extends along the medial side of the great toe and attaches to the proximal first metatarsal base.

Shim and colleagues more recently reported their experience with 8 patients with long-term follow-up between 2.3 and 13.8 years with overall acceptable results, but warned that any LEB should be identified and surgically treated to prevent recurrence. Their general guidelines recommended addressing any polydactyly; releasing the medial forefoot; correction of MTP incongruity; and treating LEB, if present. Depending on concomitant findings, excision of extranumerary bones, osteotomies, skin flaps, and soft tissue procedures were determined on an individualized basis.[1]

## CLINIC CARE POINTS

- Rare condition that causes abnormal medial varus angulation of the first metatarsal phalangeal joint and a widened enlarged first web space cleft.
- Associated with polydactyly and longitudinal epiphyseal brackets.
- Surgical treatment consists of addressing polydactyly and LEB, if present; releasing medial structures and providing soft tissue coverage via a proximal dorsal or plantar first web space rotational flap.

## OVERLAPPING FIFTH TOE

Overlapping fifth toe is also known as an overriding fifth toe, congenital fifth toe varus, crossover toe, and digiti quinti varus.[26,41–43] It is a congenital defect with no gender preference that often occurs bilaterally and can cause shoe wear difficulties, pain, and occasional disability in up to half of patients.[43–48] It is characterized by dorsal and varus angulation of a hypoplastic externally rotated small toe associated with a short extensor tendon. The fourth webspace is contracted along with the dorsomedial fifth metatarsophalangeal (MTP) joint and the surrounding soft tissue structures.[41,42,47,49] The nature of the overlapping fifth toe can range from a dynamic crossover to a fixed deformity depending on the tightness of the extensor digitorum longus (EDL) tendon and the chronicity of the abnormality. In more severe instances, the MTP joint can even subluxed or dislocated.[43,46,48]

Conservative management has been advocated in younger patients with minor symptoms using taping, strapping, bracing, shoe wear modifications, and splinting techniques.[45,50] Although long-term treatment and follow-up have been shown to be helpful with these methods, recurrence is not uncommon when treatment stops.[51,52]

For those who fail conservative management and are symptomatic, operative treatment is indicated. Classically, the Lapidus procedure described releasing the EDL distally and attaching it to the conjoint tendon of the abductor digiti minimi and FDB, thus correcting the extension, adduction, and rotational deformities using only soft tissues.[42] Similarly, Zanoli described releasing the EDL more proximally along the level of the tarsometatarsal joint and rerouting the tendon subcutaneously and attaching along the plantar surface of proximal phalanx and abductor with the toe held in realignment.[53] Both operations were based on V-to-Y advancement flaps and were complicated by scar contractures and recurrence.

Considered the "gold standard," the Butler procedure was developed using a circumferential racket type incision that provides the ability to release the extensor tendon and MTP capsule, while providing enough soft tissue mobilization and exposure to correct for contractures.[4]

Leonard recommended excising full-thickness U-shaped skin between the fourth and fifth toe web space and syndactylyzing the toes together. In this manner, the small toe is internally splinted, attached, and kept corrected next to the fourth toe at the cost of another cosmetic deformity.[54] Wound healing complications along the fourth web space have also been associated with this technique.[55]

Murgier described 16 patients treated successfully with a less invasive percutaneous-based technique adapted to the pediatric population. It avoids soft tissue complications such as scarring, recurrence, and vascular injuries associated with prior techniques requiring advancement V-Y flaps.[44]

Because of lack of good high-powered studies and lack of long-term follow-up, no technique has been proven to be superior to any other.

## CLINIC CARE POINTS

- Congenital fifth toe short extensor tendon resulting in an overlapping, angular and rotational deformity over the fourth toe with concomitant soft tissue contractures.
- Surgical treatment is offered upon failure of conservative management.
- No single operative technique, including the Butler procedure, has been proven to be most effective.

## MACRODACTYLY

Macrodactyly is a rare gross enlargement of one or more digits in the hands and feet. It can involve just the phalanges and occasionally the entire ray including the metatarsal, and is a localized form of gigantism.[56,57] Typically, the skin, bone, muscles, ligaments, neurovascular structures, and fat are all involved in the overgrowth. Most cases present at birth and may be categorized as static (proportional) enlargement as compared to the rest of the limb and surrounding digits versus progressive enlargement over time.[58,59] Hands are usually more affected than feet and are more closely associated with neural involvement.[56,57,60] The incidence is 1/50,000 to 1/100,000 live births, is unilateral in 95% of cases, and is nongender specific. Many cases, especially those with Proteus syndrome, appear to be associated with PIK3CA and AKT1 somatic gene mosaicisms.[61] The second and third toes are most commonly involved. The distal structures are more involved than the proximal ones. Occasionally, syndactyly may occur concomitantly. The nail plate's significantly enlarged and widened presence requires consideration during operative reconstruction. Fortunately, overgrowth of the digit stops upon the child's skeletal maturation (**Fig. 4**).

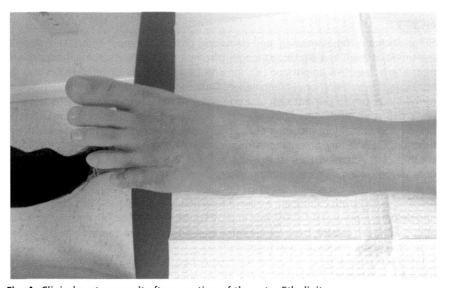

**Fig. 4.** Clinical post-op result after resection of the extra 5th digit.

The gross enlargement of the digit(s) leads to significant deformity, angular malalignment, pain, shoe wear problems, disability, and psychosocial distress—treatment is surgical through debulking procedures, selective phalangeal or ray resections, amputations, and epiphysiodesis. The diseased digits are enlarged in all dimensions, including length, height, and width. In later years, pain may develop from postoperative sequelae, degenerative changes, stiffness, and further deformity.

Hypertrophied fibrofatty proliferation accounts for the majority of the thickness and bulkiness of the enlarged toes and characteristically presents with fatty lobules intertwined with a dense, thick mesh of fibrous tissue. Histologically, there is a proliferation of fusiform cells interspersed with collagen fibers found in the subperiosteal layer overlying the cortical bone.[60]

Macrodactyly has also been known as macrosomia, dactylomegaly, macrodystrophia lipomatosa, and megalodactyly.

Although most presentations are solitary and idiopathic, this condition has been associated with:

1. Neurofibromatosis—may have a family history.
2. Proteus syndrome (multiple hamartomatous abnormalities)
3. Klippel-Trenaunay syndrome[62]

## GENETIC COUNSELING

Although the vast majority of cases are idiopathic and solitary, genetic evaluation and testing are recommended in cases where family history and/or syndromic features are present or suspected, for example, neurofibromatosis, Proteus syndrome, and other overgrowth syndromes.

## IMAGING

Serial radiographs of the affected limb help to follow and document bone and soft tissue growth over time. A preoperative CT scan of the limb is occasionally needed for surgical planning.

### Surgery

Surgical shortening, narrowing, and debulking provide the most definitive method of treatment. If there is a significant length discrepancy, phalangectomy, temporary or permanent selective epiphysiodesis (growth plate closure), or amputation may be considered in isolation or in combination. Debulking of fibrofatty tissue must be performed judicially to prevent vascular compromise or ischemia. Oanielsson reported on 3 cases of macrodactyly where they performed V-shaped resections through plantar and dorsal foot incisions of the middle toes resulting in better cosmesis and function.[63] Entire ray amputations may also be necessary to decrease the foot's width.[56,64,65] Attention to shaping and resizing the nail plate/bed should also be considered during surgical planning. Staged procedures are not uncommon as the digit continues to grow and develop. Delaying surgery can potentially limit rebound reactive overgrowth, although earlier interventions may reduce gait disturbances and deformity, prevent disability, and improve quality of life, function and psychosocial status. For each patient, treatment is individualized to achieve appropriate "shoeable" foot, correction, cosmesis, and function.[56]

Long-term follow-up is necessary because of postoperative wound complications, necrosis, degenerative changes, tissue imbalances, further deformity, and continued overgrowth, especially in younger children.

## CLINIC CARE POINTS

- Rare disorder resulting in disproportional and progressive enlargement of one or more digits in the feet causing significant disfigurement and disability.
- Surgical intervention is the mainstay treatment to shorten and debunk the affected digit.
- May have genetic link to neurofibromatosis, Proteus syndrome, and other overgrowth syndromes. In Proteus syndrome, PIK3CA and AKT1 somatic gene mosaicisms have been implicated.
- Long-term follow-up is required for conservative and surgical treatment and for postoperative complications (eg, stiffness, pain, deformity, recurrence).

## DISCLOSURE

The authors have nothing to disclose.

## REFERENCES

1. Jordan D, Hindocha S, Dhital M, et al. The epidemiology, genetics and future management of syndactyly. Open Orthop J 2012;6:14–27.
2. Kelly DM, Mahmoud K, Mauck BM. Polydactyly of the foot: a review. J Am Acad Orthop Surg 2021;29(9):361–9.
3. Nogami H. Polydactyly and polysyndactyly of the fifth toe. Clin Orthop Relat Res 1986;204:261–5.
4. Ahmed H, Akbari H, Emami A, et al. Genetic overview of syndactyly and polydactyly. Plast Reconstr Surg Glob Open 2017;5(11):e1549.
5. Adler J, Gentless J, Springer K, et al. Concomitant syndactyly and polydactyly in a pediatric foot. J Foot Ankle Surg 1997;36(2):151–4.
6. Malik S. Polydactyly: phenotypes, genetics and classification. Clin Genet 2014;85(3):203–12.
7. Frazier T. A note on race-specific congenital malformation rates. Am J Obstet Gynec 1960;80:184–5.
8. Vasluian E, van der Sluis CK, van Essen AJ, et al. Birth prevalence for congenital limb defects in the northern Netherlands: a 30-year population-based study. BMC Musculoskelet Disord 2013;14:323.
9. Castilla EE, Lugarinho R, da Graça Dutra M, et al. Associated anomalies in individuals with polydactyly. Am J Med Genet 1998;80(5):459–65.
10. Herring J, Tachdjian M. Tachdjian's pediatric orthopaedics. 6th edition. Philadelphia: Saunders/Elsevier; 2022. p. 778–9.
11. Belthur MV, Linton JD, Barnes DA. The spectrum of preaxial polydactyly of the foot. J Pediatr Orthop 2011;31(4):435–47.
12. Venn-Watson EA. Problems in polydactyly of the foot. Orthop Clin North Am 1976;7:909–27.
13. Seok HH, Park JU, Kwon ST. New classification of polydactyly of the foot on the basis of syndactylism, axis deviation, and metatarsal extent of extra digit. Arch Plast Surg 2013;40(3):232–7.
14. Turra S, Gigante C, Bisinella G. Polydactyly of the foot. J Pediatr Orthop B 2007;16(3):216–20.
15. Kubat O, Antičević D. Does timing of surgery influence the long-term results of foot polydactyly treatment? Foot Ankle Surg 2018;24(4):353–8.

16. Togashi S, Nakayama Y, Hata J, et al. A new surgical method for treating lateral ray polydactyly with brachydactyly of the foot: lengthening the reconstructed fifth toe. J Plast Reconstr Aesthet Surg 2006;59(7):752–8.
17. Langlais T, Rougereau G, Marty-Diloy T, et al. Surgical treatment in child's congenital toe syndactyly: risk factor of recurrence, complication and poor clinical outcomes [published online ahead of print, 2021 Feb 19]. Foot Ankle Surg 2021.
18. Kawabata H, Ariga K, Shibata T, et al. Open treatment of syndactyly of the foot. Scand J Plast Reconstr Surg Hand Surg 2003;37(3):150–4.
19. Hayashi A, Yanai A, Komuro Y, et al. A new surgical technique for polysyndactyly of the toes without skin graft. Plast Reconstr Surg 2004;114(2):433–8.
20. Lim YJ, Teoh LC, Lee EH. Reconstruction of syndactyly and polysyndactyly of the toes with a dorsal pentagonal island flap: a technique that allows primary skin closure without the use of skin grafting. J Foot Ankle Surg 2007;46(2):86–92.
21. Marsh DJ, Floyd D. Toe syndactyly revisited. J Plast Reconstr Aesthet Surg 2011; 64(4):535–40.
22. Aizawa T, Togashi S, Haga Y, et al. Linear separation of toe syndactyly with preserved subcutaneous vascular network skin grafts. Ann Plast Surg 2017;78(3):311–4.
23. Biyani A, Jones DA, Murray DM. Flexor to extensor tendon transfer for curly toes. Acta Orthop Scand 1992;63(4):451–4.
24. Turner PL. Strapping of curly toes in children. Aust N Z J Sur 1987;57:467–70.
25. Smith WG, Seki JT, Smith RW. Prospective study of noninvasive treatment for two common congenital toe abnormalities. Paediatr Child Health 2007;12(9):755–9.
26. Talusan PG, Milewski MD, Reach JS Jr. Fifth toe deformities - overlapping and underlapping Toe. Foot Ankle Spec 2013;10(10):1–5.
27. Sweetnam R. Congenital curly toes: an investigation into the value of treatment. Lancet 1958;11:398–400.
28. Pollard JP, Morrison PJM. Flexor tenotomy in the treatment of curly toes. Proc R Soc Med 1975;68:480–1.
29. Tokioka K, Nakatsuka T, Tsuji S, et al. Surgical correction for curly toe using open tenotomy of flexor digitorum brevis tendon. J Plast Reconstr Aesthet Surg 2007; 60:1317–22.
30. Ross ERS, Menelaus MB. Open flexor tenotomy for hammer toes and curly toes in childhood. J Bone Joint Surg Br 1984;66-B:770–1.
31. Hamer AJ, Stanley D, Smith TW. Surgery for curly toe deformity: a double-blind, randomized, prospective trial. J Bone Joint Sur Br 1993;75:662–3.
32. Taylor RG. The treatment of claw tower by multiple transfer of flexor into extensor tendons. J Bone Joint Surg Br 1951;33-B:539–42.
33. Mubarak SJ, O'Brien TJ, Davids JR. Metatarsal epiphyseal bracket; treatment by central physiolysis. J Pediatr Orthop 1993;13(1):5–8.
34. Sobel E, Levitz S, Cohen R, et al. Longitudinal epiphyseal bracket: associated foot deformities with implications for treatment. J Am Podiatry Med Assoc 1996;86(4):147–55.
35. Shim JP, Lim TK, Kyoung HK, et al. Surgical treatment of congenital hallux varus. Clinic Ortho Surg 2014;6:216–22.
36. Farmer AW. Congenital hallux varus. Am J Surg 1958;95(2):274–8.
37. Buck-Gramcko D. Congenital hallux varus. Operat Orthop Traumotol 2003;15: 463–72.
38. Mills JA, Menelaus MB. Hallux varus. J Bone Joint Surg Br 1989;71(3):437–40.
39. McElvenny RT. Hallux varus. Q Bull Northwest Univ Med Sch 1941;15:277–80.
40. Stanifer E, Hodor D, Wertheimer S. Congenital hallux varus: case presentation and review of the literature. J Foot Surg 1991;30(5):509–12.

41. Lantzounis L. Congenital subluxation fo the fifth toe and its correction by a periosteo-capsuloplasty and tendon transplantation. J Bone Joint Surg Am 1940;22:147–50.
42. Lapidus P. Transplantation of the extensor tendon for correction of the overlapping fifth toe. J Bone Joint Surg Am 1942;24:555–9.
43. Black GB, Grogan DP, Bobechko WP. Butler arthroplasty for correction of the adducted fifth toe: a retrospective study of 36 operations between 1968 and 1982. J Pediatr Ortho 1985;5:439–41.
44. Murgier J, Knorr J, Soldado F, et al. Percutaneous correction of congenital overlapping fifth toe in pediatric patients. Orthop Traumatol Surg Res 2013;99:737–40.
45. Goodwin F, Swisher F. The treatment of congenital hyperextension fo the fifth toe. J Bone Joint Surg Am 1943;25:193–6.
46. Rosner M, Knudsen HA, Sharon SM. Overlapping fifth toe: a new surgical approach. J Foot Surg 1978;17:67–9.
47. Cockin J. Butler's operation for an overriding fifth toe. J Bone Joint Surg Br 1968; 50:78–81.
48. Johnson CP, Hugar DW. A literature review of congenital digiti quinti varus: clinical description and treatment. J Foot Surg 1983;22:116–20.
49. Weber RB. Surgical criteria for correcting the overlapping fifth toe. J Foot Surg 1982;21:30–6.
50. Roven MD. A traction sling to affect an overlapping fifth toe. J AM Podiatry Assoc 1959;49:376.
51. Scrase W. The treatment of dorsal adduction deformities of the gift toe: proceedings and reports of universities, colleges, councils, and associations Great Britain. J Bone Joint Surg Br 1954;36:146.
52. Paton RW. Plasty for correction varus fifth toe. J Pediatr Ortho 1990;10:248–9.
53. de Palma L, Zanoli G. Zanoli's procedure for overlapping fifth toe:retrospective study of 18 cases followed for 14-17 years. Acta Ortho Scand 1998;69:505–7.
54. Leonard MH, Rising EE. Syndactylization to maintain correction of overlapping 5th toe. Clin Ortho Relat Res 1965;43:241–3.
55. Hulman S. Simple operation for the overlapping fifth toe. Br Med J 1964;2:1506–7.
56. Chang CH, Kumar SJ, Riddle EC, et al. Macrodactyly of the foot. J Bone Joint Surg 2002;84A:1189–94.
57. Kalen V, Burwell DS, Omer GE. Macrodactyly of the hand and feet. J Pediatr Orthop 1988;8:311–5.
58. Barsky AJ. Macrodactyly. J Bone Joint Surg 1967;49A:1255–66.
59. Dennyson WG, Bear JN, Bhoola KD. Macrodactyly in the foot. J Bone Joint Surg 1977;59B:355–9.
60. Syed A, Sherwani R, Azam Q, et al. Congenital macrodactyly: a clinical study. Acta Ortho Belg 2005;71:399–404.
61. Tian W, Huang Y, Sun L, et al. Phenotypic and genetic spectrum of isolated macrodactyly: somatic mosaicism of PIK3CA and AKT1 oncogenic variants. Orphanet J Rare Dis 2020;15:288.
62. Hop MJ, van der Biezen JJ. Ray reduction of the foot in the treatment of macrodactyly and review of the literature. J Foot Ankle Surg 2011;50:434–8.
63. Oanielsson L. Resection for macrodactylism of toes: report of three cases. Acta Orthop Scand 1986;57:560–2.
64. Kim J, Park JW, Hong SW, et al. Ray amputation for the treatment of foot macrodactyly in children. J Bone Joint Surg Br 2015;97:1364–9.
65. Dedrick D, Kling TF Jr. Ray resection in the treatment of macrodacyly of the foot in children. Orthop Trans 1985;9:145.

# Pediatric Sports Injuries

Joshua Strassberg, MD, FAAOS[a], Aamir Ahmed, DPM, AACFAS[b],*

## KEYWORDS

- Chronic exertional compartment syndrome • Exertional pain • Stress fractures
- Turf toe • Sesamoiditis • Forefoot pain • Leg pain • Repetitive stress

## KEY POINTS

- Pediatric patients are susceptible to overuse injuries in the lower leg, ankle, and foot.
- Thorough history and examination are necessary for proper diagnosis.
- Most of the overuse issues are amenable to nonoperative treatment though there are specific injuries that are treated more successfully with surgical intervention.
- Radiographic findings are normal in cases of sesamoiditis as well as grade 1 and 2 Turf toe.
- Turf toe injury from literature is known to end in long-term stiffness and pain in the affected joint.

## CHRONIC EXERTIONAL COMPARTMENT SYNDROME

A compartment syndrome is defined as a condition in which pressure increases within a confined space in the body. The increased pressure subsequently results in a decrease in the blood flow and perfusion of the tissues within that compartment, which in turn leads to ischemia and possible damage to those tissues. These conditions typically occur in the compartments containing the muscles, blood vessels, and nerves of the upper or lower extremities.

### Etiology

Compartment syndrome can be acute, as is seen in traumas such as fractures, or chronic, which may be seen with repetitive exertion. The repetitive exertion, particularly eccentric contracture of the muscle,[1] can lead to increased intramuscular and intracompartmental pressure and constriction of the perfusion of the structures within the compartment. This decreased perfusion may result in pain, which in turn limits the athlete's ability to continue with their activities. The compression of the nerves in the compartment may also lead to paresthesia or decreased sensations in the nerve's distribution distally.

[a] The Pediatric Orthopedic Center, 218 Ridgedale Avenue, Suite 101, Cedar Knolls, NJ 07927, USA; [b] Ankle and Foot Doctors of New Jersey, 225 Millburn Avenue, Suite #104B, Millburn, NJ 07041, USA
* Corresponding author.
E-mail address: aahmeddpm@gmail.com

Clin Podiatr Med Surg 39 (2022) 89–103
https://doi.org/10.1016/j.cpm.2021.08.003
podiatric.theclinics.com

## Anatomy

The most common area to find chronic exertional compartment syndrome in athletes is the lower leg and may often be seen in running and cycling sports. There are 4 compartments in the lower leg: the anterior compartment, the lateral compartment, the superficial posterior compartment, and the deep posterior compartment (**Fig. 1**). Some people consider the posterior tibialis muscle to be a separate fifth compartment. These compartments contain muscles, blood vessels, and nerves. The anterior tibial artery and deep peroneal nerve are found in the anterior compartment. The superficial peroneal nerve and lateral fibular vessels are contained in the lateral compartment. The superficial posterior compartment houses the sural nerve, whereas the deep posterior compartment holds the posterior tibial neurovascular structures as well as the peroneal vessels.

Vigorous activity can cause muscles to swell up to 20 times their resting size, increasing their volume and weight by 20%.[2] Although the muscle fibers can expand, the compartments do not. The expansion of the muscles and the lack of additional space lead to increased pressure within the muscle compartment. This increased pressure can lead to decreased arterial as well as venous blood flow, which in turn leads to ischemia and subsequent ischemic pain. The pain persists until the increased compartmental pressures drop low enough to resume adequate blood flow. As opposed to acute compartment syndrome, the muscle and nerve damage is temporary, with no long-term effects.

It is not understood why some athletes are more susceptible than others. It is thought that there are multiple anatomic factors at the root of it. Although the limited space available to contain the swollen muscles plays a role in the development of the compartment syndrome, it is unlikely that it is the sole component.[3] After compartment fascial release, the total intramuscular pressure remains elevated at rest versus normal individuals, so arteriole pressure regulation may also play a role. More than a third of patients with compartment syndrome have also been found to have fascial herniations, particularly in the anterior and lateral compartments.

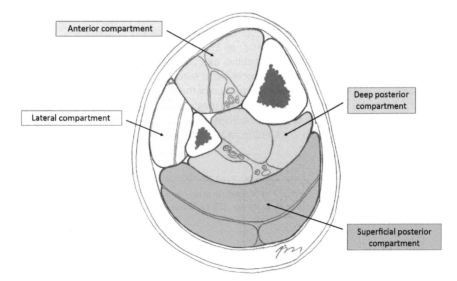

**Fig. 1.** Cross-section of the lower leg.

## Clinical Examination

Delay in diagnosis is common. Patients usually present with complaints of activity-related pain. Most patients will complain of symptoms bilaterally. The pain starts as a dull ache and progressively worsens as the athlete continues to play. The symptoms often become consistent in onset and severity of pain, starting the same amount of time into the activity. The pains classically begin approximately 10 to 15 minutes after the start of activity and resolve soon after the activity is stopped.[4] The pain is localized to the specific compartment that is affected. Numbness may also occur in the distribution of the nerve that is contained in the affected compartment. The symptoms return once activities are resumed.

The physical examination is typically unremarkable when performed at rest. The patients are neurovascularly intact. Imaging such as X ray or MRI can be used to rule out other causes of the pain but are usually negative.

## Testing

Intracompartmental pressure testing is the best method of confirming chronic exertional compartment syndrome. Pressures are typically measured before and after exercise using a needle manometer[5–8] or similar device. The criteria of Pedowitz and colleagues[5] are used for diagnosis. Positive criteria include a pre-exercise pressure greater than 15 mm Hg and a measurement taken 1 minute after exercise greater than 30 mm Hg or a 5-min post-exercise pressure greater than 20 mm Hg.

## Differential Diagnosis

The differential diagnoses include medial tibial stress syndrome, stress fractures, chronic regional pain syndrome, peripheral nerve or arterial entrapment syndromes, deep vein thrombosis, radiculopathy, or arterial vascular disease.

## Treatment Options

Chronic exertional compartment syndrome can be treated nonoperatively by eliminating or modifying the offending activity. However, few athletes are willing to modify or eliminate their activity. To eliminate the pain and still allow the patient to participate in their activity, surgical intervention is required.

Surgery entails performing fasciotomies of the affected compartments. The anterior and lateral compartments can be released through a single lateral incision or through an endoscopically assisted two-incision technique (**Fig. 2**A, B). The incision is made halfway between the tibia and fibula in longitudinal fashion. The anterior intermuscular septum is identified. A nick is made in the fascia of the anterior compartment approximately 1 cm anterior to the septum. A second nick is made in the fascia of the lateral compartment approximately 1 cm posterior to the septum, avoiding the superficial peroneal nerve. The fasciotomies are extended both proximally and distally under direct supervision. The fascia should be inspected for any herniations, which should be included in the fasciotomy. Alternatively, 2 smaller incisions can be made, one more proximal and one more distal. The subcutaneous tissues can be undermined, and the fasciotomies can be performed under endoscopic visualization.

The posterior compartments are most often accessed via a medial longitudinal incision (see **Fig. 2**C). The superficial posterior compartment can be easily released as it is directly visualized. The subcutaneous tissues can be undermined anteriorly to reach the posteromedial margin of the tibia to reach the deep posterior compartment. A specific fasciotomy of the posterior tibialis muscle is also recommended.

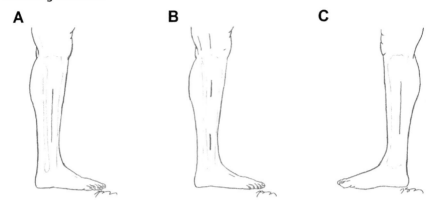

**Fig. 2.** Incisions to access the compartments of the lower leg for decompressive fasciotomies. (*A*) A longer central lateral incision can be used to access the anterior and lateral compartments. This larger incision can also be used to access the superficial and deep posterior compartments using a perifibular approach. (*B*) Two smaller lateral incisions will allow access to the anterior and lateral compartments with less soft tissue trauma. (*C*) A medial incision can be used to access the posterior compartments.

Patients may weight-bear as tolerated and begin active range of motion immediately after surgery. They may return to full activities 3 to 4 weeks postoperative.

### Outcomes

Outcomes of surgical release of the anterior and lateral compartments are high. Studies show pain improvement in 81% to 100% of patients.[9,10] Results for posterior compartment release are much less positive with success rates from 50% to 65%.[6,7,10] Recurrence rates of 7% to 17% have been reported.[6,7,10] Complication rates range from 4% to 13%[2,6,7,10] and include wound infection, hematoma/seroma, lymphocele, peripheral cutaneous nerve injury, and deep vein thrombosis.

## STRESS FRACTURES

Fractures are a common injury sustained in sports. A break in the bone can occur due to either acute trauma or excessive repetitive stress to the bone. Repetitive forces can cause small cracks in the bone which, given time, can progress on to a complete fracture.

### Etiology

Stress fractures often are due to overuse, though they can also be due to conditions that weaken the bone, such as osteoporosis. Stress fractures generally occur when the stress placed on the bone is more than the bone can handle. The bone naturally adapts to stresses gradually by remodeling, where the bone initially is resorbed and then replaced with new bone. If the increase in stress occurs too quickly, the bone cannot keep up with the need to replace the bone. If the bone is not able to keep up with the demand needed to replace the bone damage incurred by repetitive stress, there can be a disruption in the process, which can then weaken the bone and make it more susceptible to fracture.

The weight-bearing bones of the lower extremities are most commonly affected. They typically occur in areas with increased stress with impact activities or in areas with poor blood supply, which limits the bone's healing potential. Stress fractures can be seen in athletes in most sports but are most often seen in long-distance runners and military recruits who are required to march for extended periods.

There are many factors that increase the risk of developing stress fractures. Athletes who participate in high-impact activities, those that involve lots of running and jumping, are at higher risk. Sudden changes in activity level, duration, or frequency increase the risk as well. Women are at higher risk than men, particularly those who have eating disorders or abnormal or absent menses. Abnormal foot structure, such as pes planus or rigid pes cavus, can make the foot more susceptible to stress fractures. Disorders that lead to weakened bone or nutritional deficiencies put the bones at risk as well.

### Clinical Examination

As stress fractures build up over time, rather than acutely, the pain often will start off mild and gradually increase as time goes on. The pain is usually activity related though can become present without activity as the athlete continues to push through the symptoms. These often occur with a sudden increase in the amount or intensity of an activity. Physical examination typically will show tenderness over the affected bone.

### Imaging

Initial imaging usually involves plain radiographs. X-ray findings unfortunately tend to lag behind clinical symptoms. Findings, particularly in cortical bone may involve subtle periosteal reaction at the fracture site as the bone tries to heal itself. As the fracture progresses, a faint lucency may present. In cancellous bone, it may be harder to pick up early signs of a stress fracture which may present as a subtle sclerotic line in the bone. If radiographs are negative but there is a high clinical suspicion, x-rays may be repeated 2 weeks later. Additional testing such as bone scans or MRIs may be helpful as they can be more sensitive and may show results much sooner than plain radiographs. MRIs can pick up subtle marrow edema which may be the earliest sign of a stress reaction. Modern MRIs can be as sensitive and far more specific than bone scans, not to mention emit far less radiation.

### Treatment

Most stress fractures will heal uneventfully; however, the athlete is forced to miss time from sports while the bones heal. Treatment typically involves elimination of the stress. This includes activity cessation or modification. Occasionally, immobilization or weight-bearing modification may be necessary. Once the stress fracture has sufficiently healed, the athlete will be able to gradually increase activity levels to return to full sports.

Certain bones are more susceptible to stress fractures than others, including the tibia, navicular, and metatarsals.

### Tibial Shaft

Stress fractures of the tibia are more typically in the posteromedial tibia but can also be in the anterior tibial cortex. The anterior stress fractures are more concerning as the anterior tibia has a poor blood supply, which puts it at risk for delayed union or nonunion. Radiographs of anterior tibia stress fractures may present with the "dreaded black line." Because of the poor blood supply and tension at the anterior fracture site, multiple studies have shown poor results with nonoperative treatment with many patients taking up to 12 months to return to sports.[11] Borens and colleagues[12] showed improved results with anterior tension band plating and grafting, with return to sports on an average of 10 weeks. Intramedullary nailing of the tibia can also be successful.

### Tarsal Navicular

The navicular is at risk for vertical stress fractures in the central third (**Fig. 3**A). This portion of the navicular has a poor blood supply. When the foot is in equinus with axial loading, as seen in foot-strike, there is central pressure from posterior to anterior from the talar head as well as medial and lateral pressure from anterior to posterior from the medial and middle cuneiform. The combination of these stresses and poor healing ability lead to the increased risk of stress fracture.

Diagnosis of navicular stress fractures is often delayed[13,14] because patients often complain of vague ankle pain and x-rays often will not pick up the fracture until much later. On examination, the patients may have point tenderness over the dorsal aspect of the navicular. Nonoperative management with rest, immobilization, and non-weight-bearing can be successful but can take a long time.[15,16] Surgical intervention, which may speed up the healing process and return to sports, can include percutaneous or open screw fixation with or without bone grafting at the fracture site (see **Fig. 3**B–D).

### Metatarsals

The metatarsals are particularly at risk for stress fractures. This is seen often in runners or military recruits who are required to walk long distances in training. The metatarsals bear the brunt of the stress during push-off when walking or running. The second and third metatarsals, which are longer and thinner than the first metatarsal, are at higher risk. As opposed to the navicular, patients will complain of localized activity-related pain in the forefoot and will have tenderness over the affected metatarsal. These stress fractures typically occur in the midshaft. X rays are used as the initial imaging modality (**Fig. 4**). Early in the process, x-rays may be negative so if there is high clinical suspicion, an MRI may be warranted. Nonoperative treatment with activity modification and immobilization is typically successful, with or without weight-bearing restrictions.

One exception to metatarsal stress fractures is the proximal fifth metatarsal stress fracture. These occur just distal to the metaphyseal/diaphyseal junction where there is a poor blood supply. This limited blood supply can lead to delayed healing or nonunion. Nonoperative treatment is most successful with immobilization and strict non-weight-bearing for 6 weeks.[17–23] Return to sports typically occurs 12 weeks or more after initiation of treatment. Nonunions can be treated with screw fixation and bone grafting. Some recommend early surgical intervention to decrease time out of sports as well as to avoid the risk of nonunion. Early surgical fixation with a cannulated screw has been shown to provide faster healing and return to sports.[24,25]

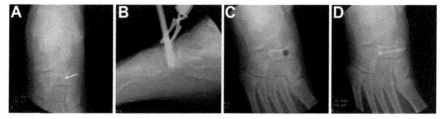

**Fig. 3.** Fluoroscopic images showing debridement and fixation of a tarsal navicular stress fracture. (*A*) The white arrow identifies the vertical stress fracture in the middle third of the navicular. (*B*) Coring the sclerotic bone at the stress fracture, directing from superior to inferior. (*C*) Following debridement of the sclerotic bone surrounding the stress. (*D*) Having been debrided and grafted with cancellous bone from the body of the calcaneus, the fracture is then compressed using a 4.0 mm headless cannulated screw.

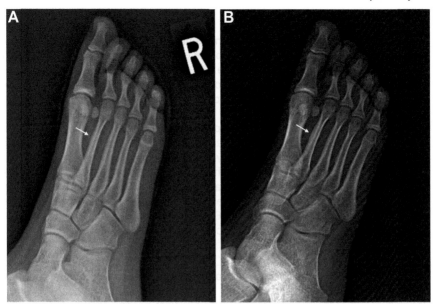

**Fig. 4.** Oblique images with white arrows showing evidence of a stress reaction in the mid-shaft of the second metatarsal. (*A*) Limited callous formation indicating early evidence of a stress fracture. (*B*) Bony callous following healing of the stress fracture.

### Prevention

Stress fractures can be prevented. There are multiple factors that lead to the development of stress fractures, including improper training methods, foot structure, and poor metabolic state. If the underlying causes of the stress fracture are not handled, the athlete may be at higher risk for delayed healing or nonunion or additional stress fractures. Patients diagnosed with stress fractures are typically tested to detect any endocrinopathies or other causes of deficiencies, particularly calcium, vitamin D, alkaline phosphatase, phosphate, and parathyroid hormone levels. Proper diet, including calcium and vitamin D, can help to strengthen the bone and reduce susceptibility to stress fractures. There are several training modifications that may help to prevent future stress fractures. Any changes to a workout regimen should occur slowly and advance gradually. Cross-training, where low-impact exercises are added, can help to decrease the trauma to one particular location. In addition, proper shoewear can help to better disperse the stress throughout the foot to reduce trauma to any one area.

### SESAMOIDITIS

Sesamoiditis is a condition that involves inflammation of the sesamoid bones that are located under the first metatarsal head due to repetitive stress or direct contusion. This is most commonly seen in young adults and teenagers.[26] This occurs mostly in athletes who are involved in running and/or vertical jumps. This is a disabling injury that can take an athlete out of the game for more than a few weeks. Certain steps can be taken to decrease the likelihood of this issue, but physicians and athletes must be educated on this topic.

### Etiology

With the latter part of gait ending in propulsion and requiring excessive stresses underneath the forefoot, there are many forefoot pathologies that can ensue. This is apparent in the population that partake in strenuous activities, such as athletes and avid runners. The final areas of pressure being underneath the first metatarsophalangeal joint and hallux during the gait cycle can result in multiple different injury types due to the many different structures involved in that area. This includes excessive and/or repetitive stresses over the sesamoid bones that lie underneath the first metatarsal head.[27]

Certain factors can increase the susceptibility of this issue. These include plantarflexed first ray, asymmetrically sized sesamoids, symmetrically enlarged sesamoids, and rotational malalignment of the first ray.[26] Although a person's anatomy and activities can play a pivotal role, it is not enough to understand the anatomy without understanding the dynamic relationship of the anatomy with the surrounding environment. Certain factors may not be anatomically related, as ground reaction forces from pavement and shoewear can also play a role. Extrinsic factors that play a role can include running surface, shoes, and extrinsic mechanical imbalances.[28]

### Anatomy and Function

Both sesamoids lie in a suspension of soft tissue combined with attachments from tendons, ligaments, and joint capsules. These structures are included in **Box 1**. Normal function of the sesamoids is to absorb weight-bearing pressure, reduce friction, and protect the Flexor Hallucis Brevis tendons during motion. They are important to the dynamic function of the first metatarsophalangeal joint and act as a fulcrum to increase the mechanical load of the Flexor hallucis brevis tendon.[27]

The sesamoids under the first metatarsal normally articulate with the first metatarsal head in their own separate grooves. The medial tibial sesamoid is usually larger than the lateral fibular sesamoid and typically has more impact during weight-bearing. This leads to higher stress and increases chances of traumatic injuries to the tibial sesamoid.[29] As the hallux dorsiflexes and plantarflexes, the position of the sesamoids changes under the metatarsal. When the first metatarsophalangeal joint dorsiflexes in closed chain movements, the motion and position of the first metatarsal can lead to greater shear and axial forces on the sesamoids along with the ground reaction forces. These are more pronounced in avid runners, sports involving vertical jumps, and activities with rapid acceleration and deceleration.[27]

### Clinical Examination

Patients typically present with an antalgic gait in acute conditions due to localized tenderness under the first metatarsal head. Localized edema and ecchymosis are

---

**Box 1**
**Structures with attachment to sesamoids**

- Flexor hallucis brevis
- Medial suspensory sesamoid ligament
- Lateral suspensory sesamoid ligament
- Medial phalangeal-sesamoidal ligament
- Lateral phalangeal-sesamoidal ligament
- Medial collateral ligament
- Lateral collateral ligament
- Deep transverse intermetatarsal ligament
- Intersesamoidal ligament

not common, but if found should raise suspicion of other significant injuries (ie, sprain, fracture). The tenderness increases on direct palpation under the first metatarsal head, and can be specific to the sesamoid location if only one sesamoid is involved. The exact location of the sesamoids and where to palpate is highlighted in **Fig. 5A, B**. The pain can also increase on dorsiflexion of the hallux or toward end dorsiflexion of the first metatarsophalangeal joint. The patient will not be able to rise on the tiptoes as they are guarding from pain.

### Imaging

Radiographic analysis in this condition is necessary to rule out a fracture or degeneration of the sesamoid complex, but will not reveal anything obvious in cases of just sesamoiditis. If the issue becomes chronic with persistent pain and failed conservative treatment for a few weeks, then a bone scan can be ordered to visualize uptake in the area of the sesamoids that can represent possible persistent inflammation. MRI is the typical advanced imaging that is obtained and can rule out persistent bone marrow inflammation or edema, stress fracture that was not visible on x-ray, avascular necrosis of the sesamoid bone, or other surrounding issues consisting of plantar plate tear, intersesamoidal ligament tear, capsulitis, or bursitis.

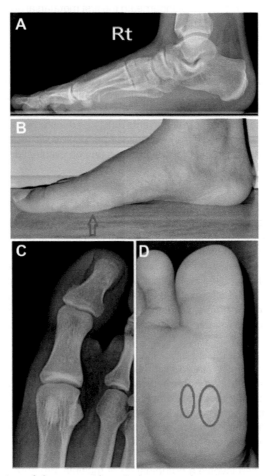

**Fig. 5.** (A–D) Location of the sesamoids and where to palpate.

### Treatment

Sesamoiditis is typically treated conservatively. Conservative management includes activity rest, ice, anti-inflammatories, activity modification, shoe modification, custom orthoses with Morton's extension to limit motion of the big toe, carbon-fiber footplate to restrict the whole forefoot motion, and/or possible cast immobilization for long periods.[27,30] When it comes to athletes, they must refrain from the sporting activity until the pain has completely resolved. This may take up to a few weeks to resolve. If pain persists and an MRI reveals persistent bone marrow edema or a stress fracture with nonunion, a bone stimulator may be used to assist with bone healing.

If conservative management has failed, surgical management may be necessitated. If a single sesamoid persists toward chronic pain, then an isolated sesamoidectomy of the symptomatic bone may be performed with caution to repair the remaining tendon and tissue and prevent an ensuing hallux valgus or varus deformity.[26]

### Prevention

Sesamoiditis may be prevented if certain early clinical signs present themselves. Owing to the injury being from repetitive stress, adequate rest for the body to heal is a crucial step. If the athlete presents with plantar forefoot pain, high arch foot type that involves a plantarflexed first ray, or callous underneath the first metatarsal head, this means there is consistently higher pressure under the forefoot. A complete foot and ankle examination must start as far back as the ankle to rule out ankle equinus. If any of the clinical or radiologic factors are apparent and that can lead to higher forces under the sesamoids, measured steps need to be taken to disperse the pressures under the foot. This can be done with simple offloading pads, gel pads, or custom orthotics. If the athlete's event requires repetitive vertical jumps (basketball, volleyball, etc.), these can be isolated traumatic events that may not be prevented as direct contusion may also lead to sesamoiditis. Athletes in these types of sporting events must be educated about the different types of injuries that can ensue and if they experience pain in specific areas, certain steps can be taken to prevent worsening of the symptoms and an eventual disabling injury.

## TURF TOE

Turf toe is a traumatic injury that results in a sprain of the plantar soft tissue structures of the first metatarsophalangeal joint. This can range in a variety of structures that can be involved. The plantar first metatarsophalangeal joint includes the capsule, sesamoidal ligaments, as well as the plantar musculature. The epidemiology is currently unknown for this injury. The only study that was performed that highlighted these values was performed specifically on collegiate football athletes. The study highlighted that the injury has an incidence of 0.062 per 1000 athletes.[31] It is mostly associated with football players because of the turf field, but can also be associated in sports such as soccer, tennis, basketball, and wrestling.[32] This can be a major cause of disability in the athlete.

### Anatomy

The structures previously stated in the sesamoiditis section are similar, except the sprained soft tissue structures are typically distal to the sesamoids. It is rare for the soft tissue structures directly proximal to the sesamoids to sustain the injury, but if they do, it is typically considered low grade. The structures distal to the sesamoids that form the plantar first metatarsophalangeal joint capsule include the plantar plate, flexor hallucis longus tendon, flexor hallucis brevis tendons, the abductor and adductor hallucis tendons, as well as parts of the medial and lateral collateral ligaments. The injury can involve a combination of multiple structures.

## Mechanism of Injury

The injury typically occurs due to hyperdorsiflexion of the first metatarsophalangeal joint in closed chain with the foot in a plantarflexed position, but can also occur with forced dorsiflexion of the hallux.[32,33] This is the typical mechanism for athletes on a turf field. Although turf field increases the friction for improved performance, friction is not known to be the greatest factor related to this issue. Rather, surface hardness and shoe flexibility have been the greatest determinants for this injury.[34] For ballet dancers, the injury occurs when the dancer falls forward over an extended toe. During normal gait, the soft tissue structures surrounding the first metatarsophalangeal joint withstand 40% to 60% of the body weight, but this can increase up to 8 times the body weight during running and jumping.[35]

## Clinical Examination

The patient will present with an antalgic gait due to pain under the big toe joint. The patient may refrain from undergoing the first metatarsophalangeal joint rocker portion of stance phase as dorsiflexion of the joint can cause pain. As with sprains of any other soft tissue structures, presentation can extend from mild to complete tear of the involved structures. Based on literature, mild sprains can be subtle, thus a high index of suspicion is warranted for these injuries.[33] Significant sprains can present with swelling, bruising, and possible paresthesia around the big toe due to traction of the surrounding nerves during injury. Palpation around the joint can specify and isolate the structures that were affected. Range of motion of the big toe joint will be limited because of guarding from pain.

## Imaging

Weight-bearing radiographic imaging must be performed as part of the initial analysis. Typical anteroposterior, lateral, and oblique views are a must and sesamoid-axial may be performed if extending the toes is tolerated by the patient. Evaluating the radiographic imaging in these injuries should involve close examination of the first metatarsal head as well as positioning of the sesamoids. The metatarsal head should be evaluated for any signs of fleck injuries that can mean possible avulsion of the capsule.[33] The sesamoids are evaluated to proximal migration or diastasis meaning tear of the plantar capsule or the intersesamoidal ligament. If proximal migration is suspected, a stress dorsiflexion radiograph can be performed under local anesthesia to evaluate the position of the sesamoids. If the sesamoids fail to track distally compared to rest position, then a plantar plate rupture can be suspected.

If the osseous structures for the most part appear normal but suspicion is still high, an MRI is commonly performed to evaluate the surrounding bone and soft tissue structures to look for tears, bone marrow edema, or loose osteochondral fragments within the first metatarsophalangeal joint.

## CLASSIFICATION

A classification was designed by Clanton and Ford in 1994 to describe the different levels of sprain and symptoms, as well as treatment strategies for each level.[36] The classification is also stressed by Anderson and colleagues with a slight modification in the treatment.

## Grade 1

This level involves a simple stretch/attenuation injury that involves minimal tearing. Clinical symptoms include plantar or medial tenderness, minimal to no ecchymosis, and minimal swelling. The athlete can typically bear weight with minimal symptoms and undergo range of motion of the first metatarsophalangeal joint with minimal restriction.

Radiographs appear normal in this grade and MRI would reveal intact soft tissue with surrounding edema.

### Grade 2

This level involves a partial tear of the plantar soft tissue structures of the first metatarsophalangeal joint. There is typically moderate swelling and ecchymosis as well as moderate tenderness on palpation. Range of motion is also restricted at the joint due to swelling and pain. The athlete will have an antalgic gait with this grade.

Radiographs can also appear normal in this grade, but MRI can demonstrate soft-tissue edema and high signal intensity deep to the plantar plate.

### Grade 3

This grade involves a complete tear of the plantar soft tissue structures at the joint. The athlete presents with an antalgic gait and clinically there is significant swelling and ecchymosis around the joint. The athlete will have severe pain, especially on range of motion of the joint. There will be weakness in flexion and instability of the joint is present.

Radiographic imaging may show sesamoid fracture, sesamoid migration proximally for one or both sesamoids, or sesamoid diastasis. If there is suspicion, a forced dorsiflexion lateral view can be taken to evaluate for sesamoid tracking and can be compared to the contralateral. MRI is beneficial in this grade as one can evaluate for complete disruption of the plantar capsule as well as possible articular impaction injuries.

## TREATMENT
### Nonoperative

The acute stages of the injury are always treated nonoperatively with rest, ice, compression, and elevation as well as anti-inflammatory medication as needed to help reduce initial pain and swelling. If the patient has an antalgic gait, they can be placed in a CAM boot, walking short leg cast, or a surgical shoe with a toe spica splint in slight plantarflexion to help immobilize the joint. For grade 1 and grade 2 injuries, taping can be used with slight plantarflexion of the joint to reduce tension on the injured tissues along with a stiff-soled shoe or a customized orthotic with a Morton's extension.[32,33] Caution must be taken with taping during the acute stages around the toe as it can reduce circulation in the toe.[35] If the medial ligamentous structures are involved and there is worry about possible traumatic hallux valgus, a toe spacer may also be inserted to prevent this issue. The difference in grade 1 and 2 is the time it takes for the acute phase with pain and inflammation to settle. An athlete with a grade 1 injury may be able to return to play with minimal pain or with a modification in shoe gear. The athlete can return as tolerated and has almost no downtime. The athlete may lose about 2 weeks of playing time with grade 2. As the acute phase starts to settle, gentle passive range of motion can begin along with low impact activities as tolerated. The athlete may progress as tolerated to full impact over the next couple week with possible conservative measures that include taping or shoe wear modification.

Grade 3 will have a similar nonoperative protocol as grades 1 and 2, but immobilization may be required for about 8 weeks. Owing to the severity of grade 3, a thorough evaluation must be performed with clinical, radiographic, and advanced imaging as acute surgical intervention has been advocated in this grade based on findings. It is recommended that the athlete's toe is protected during gradual return to full impact with taping as the deformity can progress during more strenuous activities, and for the athlete to have 50° to 60° of passive pain-free dorsiflexion before they return to play.

If the athlete has mild symptoms of pain, their shoewear can be modified with a toe turf plate or a custom orthotic with a Morton's extension. Depending on the severity of the injury, it may take a few months for the pain to completely resolve in more severe cases.

### Surgical Intervention

Surgical intervention is not advocated for grades 1 and 2, and only if specific criteria are met in grade 3 injuries. These criteria, as described by McCormick and Anderson, include large capsular avulsion with an unstable metatarsophalangeal joint, diastasis of bipartite sesamoid, diastasis of sesamoid fracture, retraction of sesamoid, traumatic hallux valgus deformity, vertical instability, loose body in the joint, chondral injury in the joint, and failed conservative management.[35] The goal is to restore the stable anatomy of the first metatarsophalangeal joint. Depending on the area of the injury, a medial J incision or dual medial and plantar lateral incisions can be used to gain access.[35]

Capsular disruption plantarly can be repaired directly end-to-end with nonabsorbable sutures while avoiding any injury to the flexor hallucis longus tendon. If the medial collateral ligaments are disrupted and a traumatic hallux valgus is evident, an adductor tenotomy is performed to balance the joint.[37]

In cases of sesamoid fractures, the smaller pole of the fracture can be removed and the remaining tissue is sutured through the larger fragment. If the fracture is too comminuted, the sesamoid can be removed, and a transfer of the abductor hallucis plantarly has been advocated to act as a plantar resistive force.[35]

Postoperative protocol requires the joint to be placed in plantarflexion and immobilized with a toe spica splint. Non-weight-bearing is performed for 4 weeks, but early gentle passive range of motion can begin at 5 to 7 days to reduce stiffness. Excessive motion should be avoided this early on. After 4 weeks, full weight-bearing can begin and active range of motion of the joint can begin as tolerated until complete range of motion is attained. At 8 weeks, a stiff-soled shoe with a turf toe plate has been recommended and the athlete can transition as tolerated into regular shoe gear with protective taping. Based on symptoms, the athlete can progress to low-impact activities to full contact.

### SEQUELAE

The injury is known from previously reported literature to end in long-term stiffness and pain in the affected joint.[32] These symptoms can take up to a year to resolve, but athletes have returned to play with this injury in modified shoe wear.

### CLINICS CARE POINTS

---

Chronic Exertional Compartment Syndrome

- Clinical suspicion is key. If chronic exertional compartment syndrome is suspected, pressure testing is necessary to make a definitive diagnosis so that proper surgical management can be performed.

Stress fractures

- Diagnosing navicular fractures may require clinical suspicion and further imaging such as a CT scan may be necessary to make the correct diagnosis.

- The location of the stress fracture in the fifth metatarsal is important in determining the risk of delayed union or nonunion and whether surgical intervention is warranted.

Sesamoiditis

- Earlier recognition of sesamoiditis and treatment increases the chances of proper healing. Having an index of suspicion will increase chances of recognition.

---

- There is a correlation between sesamoiditis and AVN. If the diagnosis is not recognized early or missed, this can result in prolonged trauma and widespread ischemia in the bone leading to AVN.
- X-ray views should include AP, oblique and sesamoid axial views. If x-ray doesn't provide enough information, MRI is commonly utilized.
- Young athletes can be eager to return to sports, but they should be counseled on the importance of initial treatment and prevention of AVN.

Turf Toe

- If turf toe injury is suspected, bilateral AP radiographs should be taken and compared to evaluate for proximal migration of the sesamoids in the symptomatic foot.
- If surgery is indicated for turf toe injury, it should be performed sooner than later as scar tissue can make proper delineation of structures difficult and can scar down a proximally retracted sesamoid complex.
- If injury is not recognized and treated properly, hallux valgus or hallux varus may ensue.

## DISCLOSURE

The authors have nothing to disclose.

## REFERENCES

1. Fronek J, Mubarak SJ, Hargens AR, et al. Management of chronic exertional anterior compartment syndrome of the lower extremity. Clin Orthop 1987;220:217–27.
2. Reneman RS. The anterior and the lateral compartmental syndrome of the leg due to intensive use of muscles. Clin Orthop 1975;113:69–80.
3. Jones DC, James SL. Overuse injuries of the lower extremity: shin splints, iliotibial band friction syndrome, and exertional compartment syndromes. Clin Sports Med 1987;6:273–90.
4. Pedowitz RA, Hargens AR, Mubarak SJ, et al. Modified criteria for the objective diagnosis of chronic compartment syndrome of the leg. Am J Sports Med 1990;18:35–40.
5. Rorabeck CH, Bourne RB, Fowler PJ. The surgical treatment of exertional compartment syndrome in athletes. J Bone Joint Surg Am 1983;65:1245–51.
6. Rorabeck CH, Fowler PJ, Nott L. The results of fasciotomy in the management of chronic exertional compartment syndrome. Am J Sports Med 1988;16:224–7.
7. Brace RA, Guyton AC, Taylor AE. Reevaluation of the needle method for measuring interstitial fluid pressure. Am J Physiol 1975;229:603–7.
8. Styf JR, Korner LM. Chronic anterior compartment syndrome of the leg: results of treatment by fasciotomy. J Bone Joint Surg Am 1986;68:1338–47.
9. Howard JL, Mohtadi NG, Wiley JP. Evaluation of outcomes in patients following surgical treatment of chronic exertional compartment syndrome in the leg. Clin J Sport Med 2000;10:176–84.
10. Friden J, Sjostrom M, Ekbolm B. Myofibrillar damage following intense eccentric exercise in man. Int J Sports Med 1983;4:170–6.
11. Torg JS, Pavlov H, Roberts MM, et al. The tarsal navicular stress fracture revisited: the unequivocal case for conservative, non-surgical management. Foot Ankle Orthop 2016;1. 2473011416S00018.
12. Khan KM, Fuller PJ, Brukner PD, et al. Outcome of conservative and surgical management of navicular stress fracture in athletes: eighty-six cases proven with computerized tomography. Am J Sports Med 1992;20:657–66.

13. Torg JS, Pavlov H, Cooley LH, et al. Stress fractures of the tarsal navicular. A retrospective review of twenty-one cases. J Bone Joint Surg Am 1982;64:700–12.
14. Gross CE, Nunley JA. Navicular stress fractures. Foot Ankle Int 2015;36:1117–22.
15. DeLee JC, Evans JP, Julian J. Stress fracture of the fifth metatarsal. Am J Sports Med 1983;11:349–53.
16. Porter DA, Rund AM, Dobslaw R, et al. Comparison of 4.5- and 5.5-mm cannulated stainless steel screws for fifth metatarsal jones fracture fixation. Foot Ankle Int 2009;30:27–33.
17. Borens O, Sen MK, Huang RC, et al. Anterior tension band plating for anterior tibial stress fractures in high- performance female athletes: a report of 4 cases. J Orthop Trauma 2006;20(6):425–30.
18. Batt ME, Kemp S, Kerslake R. Delayed union stress fractures of the anterior tibia: conservative management. Br J Sports Med 2001;35(1):74–7.
19. Torg JS, Balduini FC, Zelko RR, et al. Fractures of the base of the fifth metatarsal distal to the tuberosity: classification and guidelines for non-surgical and surgical management. J Bone Joint Surg Am 1984;66(2):209–14.
20. Shindle M, Endo Y, Warren R, et al. Stress fractures about the tibia, foot, and ankle. J Am Acad Orthop Surg 2012;20:167–76.
21. Boden B, Osbahr D. High-risk stress fractures: evaluation and treatment. J Am Acad Orthop Surg 2000;8:344–53.
22. Patel K, Christopher Z, Hubbard C, et al. Stress fractures of the fifth metatarsal in athletes. J Am Acad Orthop Surg 2021;00:1–11.
23. Garcia-Mata S, Hidalgo-Overjero A, Martinez-Grande M. Chronic exertional compartment syndrome of the legs in adolescents. J Ped Orthop 2001;21:328–34.
24. Fraipont M, Adamson G. Chronic exertional compartment syndrome. J Am Acad Orthop Surg 2003;11:268–76.
25. Pell R, Khanuja H, Cooley G. Leg pain in the running athlete. J Am Acad Orthop Surg 2004;12:396–404.
26. Boike A, Schnirring-Judge M, McMillin S. Sesamoid disorders of the first metatarsophalangeal joint. Clin Podiatric Med Surg 2011;28(2):269–85.
27. Richardson EG. Injuries to the hallucal sesamoids in the athlete. Foot Ankle 1987;7(4):229–44.
28. Richardson GE. Hallucal sesamoid pain: causes and surgical treatment. J Am Acad Orthop Surg 1999;7(4):270–8.
29. Lillich JS, Baxter DE. Common forefoot problems in runners. Foot & Ankle 1986;7(3):145–51.
30. Aiyer A, Hennrikus W. Foot pain in the child and adolescent. Pediatr Clin North Am 2014;61(6):1185–205.
31. George E, Harris AH, Dragoo JL, et al. Incidence and risk factors for turf toe injuries in intercollegiate football. Foot Ankle Int 2013;35(2):108–15.
32. Anderson R. Turf toe injuries of the hallux metatarsophalangeal joint. Tech Foot Ankle Surg 2002;1(2):102–11.
33. Bowers KD Jr, Martin RB. Turf-toe: a shoe-surface related football injury. Med Sci Sports 1976;8(2):81–3.
34. McCormick JJ, Anderson RB. Turf toe: anatomy, diagnosis, and treatment. Sports Health 2010;2(6):487–94.
35. McCormick JJ, Anderson RB. The great toe: failed turf toe, chronic turf toe, and complicated sesamoid injuries. Foot Ankle Clin 2009;14(2):135–50.
36. Clanton TO, Ford JJ. Turf toe injury. Clin Sports Med 1994;13(4):731–41.
37. Clough TM, Majeed H. Turf toe injury - current concepts and an updated review of literature. Foot Ankle Clin 2018;23(4):693–701.

# Pediatric Osteochondritis Dissecans of the Talus

Mark J. Mendeszoon, DPM[a],*, Hayley E. Iosue, DPM, AACFAS[b]

## KEYWORDS

- Pediatric • Osteochondral dissecans • Talus • Defect • Adolescent

## KEY POINTS

- OCDs should be a differential diagnosis in ankle injuries in the pediatric population .
- It is important to recognize OCDs early in the pediatric population to avoid future complications.
- The major presenting complaints in the pediatric population with a OCD are pain, stiffness, and swelling.
- Various treatment options, including conservative and surgical, are warranted in patients with pediatric OCD.

## INTRODUCTION

Konnig first described osteochondral dissecans (OCD) in the knee in 1888 as a subchondral inflammatory process. In 1922, Kappis described this condition in the talus. Juvenile osteochondritis dissecans of the talus is a rare condition in this subset of population, thus literature on this condition is minimal.[1] It involves an initial idiopathic injury to the subchondral bone of the talus that can eventually progress to the injury of the articular cartilage. Early recognition and conservative treatment are the primary treatment protocol followed by surgical intervention if a patient does not respond favorably to noninvasive treatment. OCD should not be confused with acute osteochondral fractures, which are typically acute injury.

## EPIDEMIOLOGY

After the knee and elbow, the ankle is the third most frequently affected joint that involves OCD's. Ankle OCD cases represent 4% of all cases.[2] In the pediatric population, a study including 85 patients with OCDs of the ankle, Kessler and colleagues concluded that female patients have a higher incidence than male patients for OCD's of the ankle. They also found that teenagers had a higher prevalence of

[a] Podiatric Surgery, University Hospitals Regional Hospitals Advanced Foot and Ankle Surgery Fellowship, Richmond Heights, OH, USA; [b] University Hospitals Richmond Medical Center, 27100 Chardon Road, Richmond Heights, OH 44143, USA
* Corresponding author. 150 Seventh Avenue, Suite 200, Chardon, OH 44024.
*E-mail address:* dr1zoom@roadrunner.com

Clin Podiatr Med Surg 39 (2022) 105–111
https://doi.org/10.1016/j.cpm.2021.09.005
0891-8422/22/© 2021 Elsevier Inc. All rights reserved.

OCDs than other pediatric age groups.[3] Patients with increased BMI are also at higher risk. Multiple studies have shown that the location of the lesion is more commonly found to occur at the medial talus similar to what is seen in adults. These medial lesions will typically involve the posterior or central portion of the talus.[3] Typically, pediatric patients do not recall an acute traumatic injury but an insidious onset of ankle pain, edema, or stiffness.

## ETIOLOGY

Multiple etiologies for juvenile OCD's have been theorized; however, no theory has been universally accepted. Microtrauma is the precipitating factor to cause OCD of the talus.[4] As there is typically no acute, traumatic injury noted, most children will continue to be active and spontaneous healing will take place over a short period of time. Those rare cases whereby the talus does not heal and the ankle joint undergoes continuous, repetitive motion and microtrauma will result in stiffness, edema, and pain. This injury progresses to disturb the blood supply to the injured talus creating sclerosis of the bone. With further stress applied to the affected area, the overlying hyaline cartilage of the talus will deteriorate and develop an osteochondral lesion and in some instances progress to osteoarthritis. If these nonhealing lesions result in damage to the articular cartilage and the fragment becomes loose or displaced, the vascularity of this fragment will be limited which can severely inhibit healing.[5,6]

## ANATOMIC CONSIDERATIONS

The talus is a unique bone not only with its unusual shape and lack of muscle attachments but also due to its marginal circulation. Blood supply to the talus is primarily supported by the posterior tibial artery, then the anterior tibial artery and peroneal artery (**Fig. 1**). The talus is a compact, hard bone primarily covered with cartilage. Five

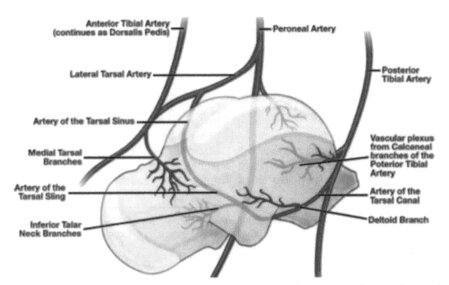

**Fig. 1.** Blood supply to the talus. (Hood CR Jr, Miller JR, Hollinger JK. Defining Talar Head and Neck Pathology: The Malvern Classification System. *J Foot Ankle Surg.* 2018;57(1):131 to 139. https://doi.org/10.1053/j.jfas.2017.07.008.)

sides of the talus are covered with cartilage and the bone contributes to the tibiotalar, subtalar, and talonavicular joints. All 3 joints have a significant impact on foot and ankle biomechanics.

The talar dome is positioned below between the medial malleolus and distal fibula. This bone is positioned between the medial and lateral malleoli. The ankle joint is supported by medial deltoid ligament, lateral ankle collateral ligaments, syndesmosis, and the distal tibiofibular ligaments. The anterior process of the talus is wider than the posterior portion of the talus and thus when the ankle is in dorsiflexion this crural joint is more stable opposed to plantarflexion.

## BIOMECHANICS OF ANKLE MOTION

The ankle joint is a hinged joint and although considered to have only a sagittal plane of motion, it actually has a complex multi-axial range of motion. This is due to the internal rotation that occurs during dorsiflexion, and the external rotation that occurs in plantarflexion. Thus, when osteochondral lesions develop, medial and lateral lesions are the 2 most common locations. Dorsiflexion-inversion injuries create a shallow anterior-lateral lesion (DIAL) and plantarflexion-inversion injuries create a deeper posterior-medial lesion. (PIMP).[7]

## CLINICAL PRESENTATION

Most pediatric patients will present initially with generalized joint pain with activity. Pain is the predominant presenting complaint in children with an OCD.[4,8] Perumal found that 97% of patients complain of pain in the ankle with an OCD. It is imperative to obtain a thorough history and physical to appreciate and investigate the activity that may have precipitated this injury. If the lesion does not spontaneously heal, the joint pain will continue to persist or worsen with activity and eventually the ankle joint will become stiff and swollen. Range of motion will become guarded and compensation of the ankle joint will ensue. Rarely does a catching or clicking sensation present like a torn meniscus in the knee present. If a loose body is present, the patient may experience locking or catching sensation during ankle joint range of motion.[4,9]

## DIAGNOSTIC WORK-UP

If an OCD is suspected during the examination, initial imaging should include AP, MO, and lateral radiographs of the ankle to evaluate for a defect. It is imperative that the treating physician appreciate the mechanism of injury and thoroughly evaluate the radiographs personally for a lesion on the talus. If a more detailed view of the OCD is warranted, an MRI can be obtained. MRI is considered the gold standard in imaging for juvenile OCD of the talus and is found to be very accurate with a sensitivity of 92% and specificity of 5%.[10] MRI evaluation can be used to better assess the overlying articular cartilage, disease progression, and possible loosening of the fragment.[2,4,8] An MRI can give a false-positive result when evaluating the instability of a lesion, so in these cases, a CT scan may be useful. CT imaging allows for better evaluation of the subchondral bone and could assist more with surgical planning.[10]

## TREATMENT

The Berndt-Hardy classification (**Fig. 2**) for adult osteochondral lesions has been adapted and used for juvenile osteochondritis dissecans of the talus. Lesions in the pediatric population have a high rate of spontaneous healing.[6] The goal of the management of these defects is to preserve the articular cartilage and heal the associated

| Stage | Description |
|---|---|
| I | Subchondral compression fracture |
| IIa | Chondral fracture (partial avulsion) |
| IIb | Subchondral cyst |
| III | Chondral fracture with separated segment (non-displaced) |
| IV | Chondral fracture with separated segment (displaced) |

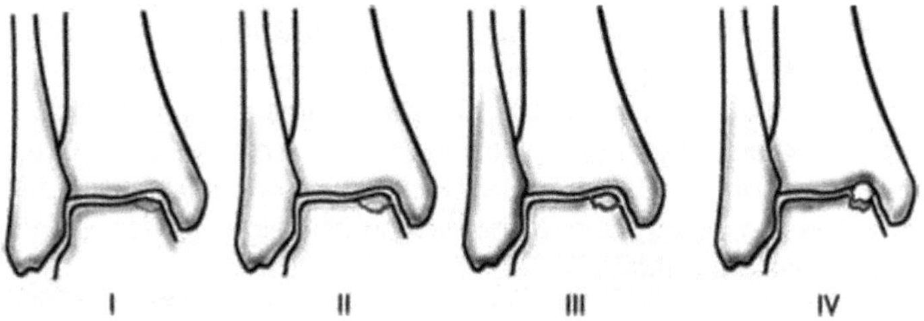

Fig. 2. Berndt Hardy Classification system and depiction.

damage as soon as possible. For juvenile osteochondritis dissecans of the talus, there are very little clear management guidelines within the literature.

## CONSERVATIVE TREATMENT

Conservative treatment options should be considered for all stable lesions and partially stable lesions in the pediatric and adolescent patient population. Nonoperative treatment modalities include cast immobilization, non–weight-bearing ankle joint range of motion, protected weight bearing, and activity modification. Many studies suggest a conservative treatment protocol of at least 6 weeks in a non–weight-bearing cast followed by 3 months of nonweight bearing but allowing for active range of motion.[4,8,9]

The success rates of various studies of conservative management vary greatly. Conservative treatment was used by Higuera and colleagues in 68% of their patient population in the study with a 94.8% success rate with outcomes being good to excellent.[8] Letts and colleagues reported that 42% of their patients with OCDs were treated conservatively and their outcomes were reported as 59% good and 38% fair.[4] Perumal and colleagues treated 59% of their patients conservatively and found 91% of patients without pain at extended follow-up.[9] Heyes and colleagues found that 61% of their patient population failed conservative treatment. They also concluded that increased patient age and grade III lesions were negative predictive factors for conservative treatment. Generally, they also found that functionally high-grade lesions would have an inferior outcome.[11]

Another treatment option to consider before or in adjunct to surgical intervention is regenerative medicine. Platelet-rich plasma (PRP) as defined as plasma with double the platelet concentration above the standard baseline $1.1 \times 10^6$ platelets/$\mu$L.[12] PRP can be useful in the treatment of a pediatric OCD due to its role in healing and it may assist with cartilage repair. PRP has been shown to cause mesenchymal stem cells to go through chondrogenic differentiation with increased type II collagen in the joint. They have also been shown to improve the cartilaginous infill via chondrocyte proliferation and mesenchymal stem cells decreasing the chance of subchondral cyst formation. (Kruger and colleagues) Many growth factors found within platelets can improve the environment for which cartilage can heal and decrease the inflammatory processes within the joint that contains an OCD.[12] In addition to PRP, the use of human amniotic tissue allograft has shown promising healing potential in patients with OCDs.[13]

## SURGICAL TREATMENT

As most osteochondral dissecan lesions in the pediatric population respond favorably to conservative treatment options, a small percentage of cases will need surgical intervention. Surgery for osteochondral lesions can be considered into 2 categories: lesion salvage and lesion excision procedures. The size of the lesion is the determining factor of which initial procedure is indicated and what procedure would be in the patient's best long-term interest and outcome. 150 mm2 is the benchmark size that would predict the outcome.[14] Chuckpaiwong and colleagues had 100% excellent surgical results in lesions smaller than 150mm2, whereas 96% of patients had a bad outcome with lesions greater than 150mm2. In addition, it is a priority to determine if a lesion is contained within the surface area of the talar dome or if the lesion is uncontained and extending into the shoulders of the talus which can be determined with advanced imaging.

Lesion salvage procedures include arthroscopic joint debridement with microfracture or drilling of the lesion. If the lesion is unstable and irreparable then excision of the lesion with transarticular drilling or microfracture is suggested. If the lesion is stable then internal fixation with an appropriately sized bioabsorbable implant is required. Typically lesion salvage procedures are initially indicated and performed on the pediatric patient.[15]

Drilling and microfracturing both disrupt intraosseous vessels which promote angiogenesis which then promotes growth factors. In time, the growth factors develop bone marrow cells which in end create a fibrocartilage substitute to form as a substitute of hyaline cartilage. The fibrocartilage that will develop will be softer than the original hyaline cartilage.[5]

Although drilling and microfracture both can stimulate a fibrocartilage plug there is a difference between the 2 techniques. It cannot be overstated that the importance of the osteochondral defect be less than 150 mm2. Lesions larger than 150 mm2 have a poor outcome with lesion salvage procedures.[16] Heat necrosis can be present with drilling and this can lead to pain, edema, stress fractures, and stiffness. Microfracturing does not causes heat necrosis but can create loose particles and if not removed may impede healing and even cause limited and painful motion.[16]

In some cases, fetal particulated articular cartilage cells can be distributed and formed into the shape of the lesion and secured with a fibrin glue.[17] In the knee, matrix-induced autologous chondrocyte implantation (MACI) has been used with some success and recently has been infrequently used in the ankle with promising results.[18] The last lesion salvage procedure is subchondroplasty of the talus. Subchondroplasty is a minimally invasive procedure that is, performed to specifically repair chronic bone marrow lesions by filling them with a bone substitute material such as a calcium phosphate or magnesium phosphate material. The bone substitute is then slowly resorbed and replaced with healthy bone, repairing the bone defect. Subchondroplasty also resolves the associated edema. Subchondroplasty may be performed alone or along with other arthroscopic procedures.

Lesion excision procedures are best indicated for unstable lesions, lesions on the shoulders of the talus, and lesions greater than 150mm2. Osteochondral autologous transplants (OATS) are performed by obtaining a cartilaginous bone harvest through obtaining multiple small grafts (mosaicplasty) or a singular cylindrical larger graft. Typically, the graft is harvested from the non–weight-bearing portion of the ipsilateral femoral condyle of the knee. The advantage of using autograft is that the incorporation of the graft should incorporate quicker than an allograft and there will be less of a host reaction of the graft than cadaveric osteochondral graft. The disadvantage is that as the knee is a large weight-bearing surface, pain and stiffness may develop as cystic changes can develop due to chondral incongruence of the surface area of the donor site. The author (MM) has avoided comorbidities at the knee site by harvesting nonweight-bearing talus autograft from the ipsilateral foot and backfilling with allograft bone or bone substitute matter.[19]

If lesions are significantly large, unstable and if lesion salvage procedures fail, then en bloc talus allografts may be successful to salvage the talus and postpone or prevent end-stage procedures such as tibio-talar arthrodesis, 3D printed talus placement, or total ankle replacement procedures.

## SUMMARY

When dealing with pediatric ankle injuries including ankle sprains, the treating physician should always include OCD as a differential diagnosis. Early recognition and conservative treatment options are paramount to the long-term health of the child's ankle. In situations that may require surgical intervention, it is important to appreciate diagnostic testing such as radiographs and MRI so that the proper surgical protocol can be provided.

## DISCLOSURE

The authors have nothing to disclose.

## REFERENCES

1. Hannon CP, Smyth NA, Murawski CD, et al. Osteochondral lesions of the talus: aspects of current management. Bone Joint J 2014;96-B(2):164–71.
2. Bruns J, Behrens P. Osteochondrosis dissecans. Arthroskopie 1998;11:166–76.
3. Kessler JI, Weiss JM, Nikizad H, et al. Osteochondritis dissecans of the ankle in children and adolescents: demographics and epidemiology. The Am J Sports Med 2014;42(9):2165–71.
4. Letts M, Davidson D, Ahmer A. Osteochondritis dissecans of the talus in children. J Pediatr Orthop 2003;23(5):617–25.
5. Vannini F, Cavallo M, Baldassarri M, et al. Treatment of juvenile osteochondritis dissecans of the talus: current concepts review. Joints 2015;2(4):188–91.
6. Bauer RS, Ochsner PE. Zur Nosologie der Osteochondrosis dissecans der Talus-rolle [Nosology of osteochondrosis dissecans of the trochlea of the talus]. Z Orthop Ihre Grenzgeb 1987;125(2):194–200.
7. Zengerink M, Struijs PA, Tol JL, et al. Treatment of osteochondral lesions of the talus: a systematic review. Knee Surg Sports Traumatol Arthrosc 2010;18(2): 238–46.
8. Higuera J, Laguna R, Peral M, et al. Osteochondritis dissecans of the talus during childhood and adolescence. J Pediatr Orthop 1998;18(3):328–32. PMID: 9600558.

9. Perumal V, Wall E, Babekir N. Juvenile osteochondritis dissecans of the talus. J Pediatr Orthop 2007;27(7):821–5.

10. Heywood CS, Benke MT, Brindle K, et al. Correlation of magnetic resonance imaging to arthroscopic findings of stability in juvenile osteochondritis dissecans. Arthroscopy 2011;27(2):194–9.

11. Heyse TJ, Schüttler KF, Schweitzer A, et al. Juvenile osteochondritis dissecans of the talus: predictors of conservative treatment failure. Arch Orthop Trauma Surg 2015;135(10):1337-41. doi:10.1007/s00402-015-2260-4.

12. Smyth NA, Murawski CD, Haleem AM, et al. Establishing proof of concept: platelet-rich plasma and bone marrow aspirate concentrate may improve cartilage repair following surgical treatment for osteochondral lesions of the talus. World J Orthop 2012;3(7):101–8.

13. Anderson J, Swayzee Z. The use of human amniotic allograft on osteochondritis dissecans of the talar dome: a comparison with and without allografts in arthroscopically treated ankles. Surg Sci 2015;6:412–7.

14. Chuckpaiwong B, Berkson EM, Theodore GH. Micro-fracture for osteochondral lesions of the ankle: outcome analysis and outcome predictors of 105 cases. Arthroscopy 2008;24:106–12.

15. Kramer DE, Glotzbecker MP, Shore BJ, et al. Results of surgical management of osteochondritis dissecans of the ankle in the pediatric and adolescent population. J Pediatr Orthop 2015;35(7):725–33.

16. Choi WJ, Jo J, Lee JW. Osteochondral lesion of the talus: prognostic factors affecting the clinical outcome after arthroscopic marrow stimulation technique. Foot Ankle Clin 2013;18(1):67–78.

17. Farr J, Cole BJ, Sherman S, et al. Particulated articular cartilage: CAIS and De-Novo NT. J Knee Surg 2012;25(1):23–9.

18. Ronga M, Grassi FA, Montoli C, et al. Treatment of deep cartilage defects of the ankle with matrix-induced autologous chondrocyte implantation (MACI). Foot Ankle Surg 2005;11(1):29–33.

19. Mendeszoon M, Wilson N, Avramaut K, Rodrigues R, et al. Surgical Correction of OCD utilizing OATS procedure harvested from head of the talus. North Ohio Foot Ankle J 2015;2(9):2.

# Assessment of Pediatric Limb Length Inequality

Jacob Wynes, DPM, MS[a],*, Alexis Schupp, DPM[b]

## KEYWORDS

- Limb length • Deformity • Alignment • Height • Malalignment

## KEY POINTS

- Ensuring appropriate and objective assessment of limb length are paramount in the management of limb length inequality.
- It is important to recognize various confounding factors that could affect limb length, such as soft tissue contractures and musculoskeletal deformity, which could result from post-traumatic or congenital influences.
- A correlation between what is observed clinically through comprehensive physical examination and radiographically should be present when assessing limb length inequality.
- Conservative and surgical means of correction to avoid abnormal compensatory kinematics are possible in the management of limb length inequality.

## INTRODUCTION

Limb length inequality or discrepancy (LLD) occurs when there is a difference in length between 2 limbs or when deviation exists from a normally expected length for a given age (**Table 1**). The magnitude of the discrepancy is defined as the difference between the 2 extremities.[1] In the rare instances both limbs are found to be affected, such as rhizomelic, mesomelic, and acromelic cases of congenital short stature. In these cases, the comparison can be made with normal length in a population for that particular age. These values historically have been published in print and now have various smart applications available for assessment and reference.[2–5] Aside from congenital etiologies, LLD can also arise from infection, paralysis, tumors/neoplasm, and surgery. Approximately 70% to 90% of the world's population has some elements of LLD with compensation allowing for tolerance and potentially masking the extent to which one limb could be significantly shorter either functionally or structurally.[6,7] Components of functional LLD could include congenital shortening of soft tissues, joint contractures, axial skeleton malalignment, and abnormal pedal biomechanics (ie, posterior tibial tendonitis or equinovarus). In accordance with literature reports, most individuals

[a] Department of Orthopaedics, University of Maryland School of Medicine, University of Maryland Limb Preservation and Deformity Correction Fellowship, 2200 Kernan Drive, Baltimore, MD 21207, USA; [b] University of Maryland Limb Preservation and Deformity Correction Fellowship, 2200 Kernan Drive, Baltimore, MD 21207, USA
* Corresponding author.
*E-mail address:* jwynes@som.umaryland.edu

Clin Podiatr Med Surg 39 (2022) 113–127
https://doi.org/10.1016/j.cpm.2021.09.004
0891-8422/22/Published by Elsevier Inc.

podiatric.theclinics.com

can tolerate upwards of a 2 cm discrepancy. Although a constellation of symptoms such as joint pain, arthritis, alterations in oxygen consumption/heart rate, and low back pathology can occur later on in adulthood, the focus in this review will be with early diagnosis and management in the pediatric population.

## LIMB LENGTH ASSESSMENT
### Clinical Evaluation

First, a thorough history is important to understand the causes of limb length discrepancy as posttraumatic and congenital influences often play a role. Additionally, an awareness of fixed scoliosis and pelvic tilt needs to be considered this may be a perception of LLD by the patient themselves. Various methods of measurement exist with varying degrees of inter-rater reliability and reproducibility.[8,9] There are 2 common ways to measure total limb length on a patient. The first is by using a measuring tape to measure the distance from the anterior superior iliac spine to the tip of the medial malleolus. The second is the measurement of the umbilicus or xiphoid to the medial malleolus. On occasion, there is no difference between measurements of each limb. This is called Apparent LLD. This is often due to fixed pelvic obliquity from spinal or hip pathology influencing these results (**Fig. 1**).

| Table 1 Lower extremity multiplier table | | | | | | | |
|---|---|---|---|---|---|---|---|
| **Boys** | | | | **Girls** | | | |
| Age (y+m) | Multiplier | Age (y+m) | Multiplier | Age (y+m) | Multiplier | Age (y+m) | Multiplier |
| Birth | 5.080 | 7 + 6 | 1.520 | Birth | 4.630 | 7 + 6 | 1.370 |
| 0 + 3 | 4.550 | 8 + 0 | 1.470 | 0 + 3 | 4.155 | 8 + 0 | 1.330 |
| 0 + 6 | 1.050 | 8 + 6 | 1.420 | 0 + 6 | 3.725 | 8 + 6 | 1.290 |
| 0 + 9 | 3.600 | 9 + 0 | 1.380 | 0 + 9 | 3.300 | 9 + 0 | 1.260 |
| 1 + 0 | 3.240 | 9 + 6 | 1.340 | 1 + 0 | 2.970 | 9 + 6 | 1.220 |
| 1 + 3 | 2.975 | 10 + 0 | 1.310 | 1 + 3 | 2.750 | 10 + 0 | 1.190 |
| 1 + 6 | 2.825 | 10 + 6 | 1.280 | 1 + 6 | 2.600 | 10 + 6 | 1.160 |
| 1 + 9 | 2.700 | 11 + 0 | 1.240 | 1 + 9 | 2.490 | 11 + 0 | 1.130 |
| 2 + 0 | 2.590 | 11 + 6 | 1.220 | 2 + 0 | 2.390 | 11 + 6 | 1.100 |
| 2 + 3 | 2.480 | 12 + 0 | 1.180 | 2 + 3 | 2.295 | 12 + 0 | 1.070 |
| 2 + 6 | 2.385 | 12 + 6 | 1.160 | 2 + 6 | 2.200 | 12 + 6 | 1.050 |
| 2 + 9 | 2.300 | 13 + 0 | 1.130 | 2 + 9 | 2.125 | 13 + 0 | 1.030 |
| 3 + 0 | 2.230 | 13 + 6 | 1.100 | 3 + 0 | 2.050 | 13 + 6 | 1.010 |
| 3 + 6 | 2.110 | 14 + 0 | 1.080 | 3 + 6 | 1.925 | 14 + 0 | 1.000 |
| 4 + 0 | 2.000 | 14 + 6 | 1.060 | 4 + 0 | 1.830 | | |
| 4 + 6 | 1.890 | 15 + 0 | 1.040 | 4 + 6 | 1.740 | | |
| 5 + 0 | 1.820 | 15 + 6 | 1.020 | 5 + 0 | 1.660 | | |
| 5 + 6 | 1.740 | 16 + 0 | 1.010 | 5 + 6 | 1.580 | | |
| 6 + 0 | 1.670 | 16 + 6 | 1.010 | 6 + 0 | 1.510 | | |
| 6 + 6 | 1.620 | 17 + 0 | 1.000 | 6 + 6 | 1.460 | | |
| 7 + 0 | 1.570 | | | 7 + 0 | 1.430 | | |

*From* Paley D, Pfeil J. Prinzipien der kniegelenknahen Deformitätenkorrektur [Principles of deformity correction around the knee]. Orthopade. 2000 Jan;29(1):18-38. German. doi: 10.1007/s001320050004. PMID: 10663243.

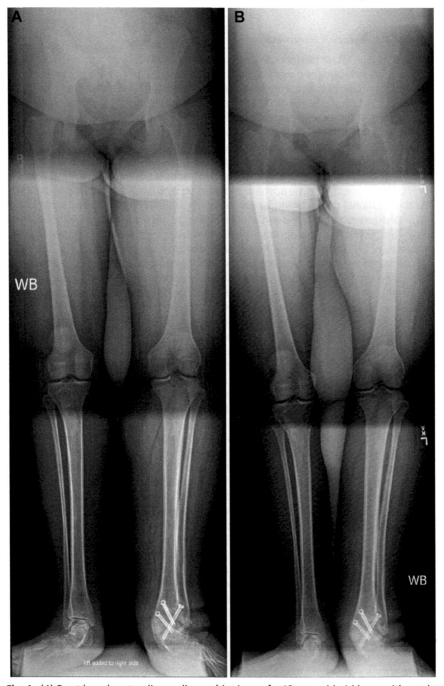

**Fig. 1.** (*A*) Erect long leg standing radiographic views of a 13-year-old girl born with myelomeningocele and <u>apparent</u> right limb length discrepancy. Measurements of left and right tibial segments reveal 38 cm and 37 cm, respectively. Measurements of the left and right femoral segments reveal 44 cm and 45 cm, respectively. Equal length of 82 cm bilateral is established with a component of pelvic obliquity that cannot be excluded. (*B*) Without lift placed demonstrating the LLD.

### Imaging/Radiographic Interpretation

In an effort to mitigate the inconsistency associated with clinical tape measure, radiographic LLD assessment remains a reliable and reproducible means of measurement. In particular, much of the interpretation has evolved through the use of picture archiving and communication systems (PACS). Plain film radiography (X-ray) and computed tomography (CT) are often incorporated as scanograms whereby the patient is usually positioned supine and 3 separate exposures are stitched onto one film from the hip, knee, and ankle. It has been shown that these images produce limited magnification artifacts as each image is centered on the joint. Images can be taken with either long or short films. Care should be taken with short film radiographs as alignment cannot effectively be measured.[10-12] One advantage conferred by CT imaging is that one can calculate the rotational profile of the femur and tibia extremities in a manner correlative of physical examination parameters (ie, thigh foot angle assessment for external tibial torsion). Tokarowski and colleagues in 1995 were able to demonstrate a higher degree of sensitivity of CT over traditional X-rays, MRI, and ultrasound.[13]

For pediatrics, a 3-foot cassette can be used to capture both lower extremities. For this, an optimal distance between the X-ray source and film is 10 feet or 305 cm centered at the knee joint with the patella pointing forward. Positioning should also include a calculated lift on the shorter extremity. The lift should be added in 1 cm incremental blocks until the level of the pelvis is equal on both sides. Of note, a distance of 10 feet leads to approximately 5% magnification.[1] Paley and colleagues estimated a total error of 1.5 mm resolved by the assumption that differences should be no greater than 2–3 cm. Thereby calculating 5% × 30 mm = 1.5 mm. The authors here recommend the incorporation of a standard magnification ball of 25.4 mm or 2.54 cm as a means of providing a more accurate assessment for LLD.

Measurements are performed by assessing the distance from the proximal most point of the 2 femoral heads to the top of the film or grid lines (as available). This measurement is then added to the height of the lifts as applicable for total limb length inequality. The use of teleorentgenogram (usually taken at a distance of 6 feet) allows for the accurate assessment of foot height and pelvic height as potential confounding factors for limb length inequality. Additionally, one should consider whether or not pelvic osteotomies/fractures, a previously dislocated hip, or femoral avascular necrosis has occurred. To account for these pathologies, other landmarks are recommended for evaluation such as the inferior pole of the sacroiliac joint. The authors do not recommend using the superior portions of the iliac crests or the inferior aspect of the ischial tuberosities as this can be a less reliable measurement in the setting of hypoplasia.

The authors of this manuscript believe a thorough and reproducible means of calculating LLD is in the following parameters set by the International Center for Limb Lengthening (ICLL) group at Sinai Hospital in Baltimore, MD. Several methods are outlined in their approach. First, with respect to total LLD, they begin by drawing 2 lines on the inferior aspect of each SI joint and drawing a pelvic line. The total LLD is calculated by the numeric measurement above using the formula: Total LLD = Short Segment + Long Segment + Height of Blocks. For the analysis of individual segments, this is carried out at the respective joint lines: femoral-acetabular, knee, and ankle. Finally, a calculation can be performed to assess either the foot segment (arch height) contribution or the length loss in the shortened limb of interest. This is calculated by adding the total LLD to the combined (change in pelvic segments + change in femoral segments + change in tibial segments) (**Fig. 2**).

One can determine the final length after angular deformity correction by calculating the length gained after surgical reconstruction. This is accomplished by adding the

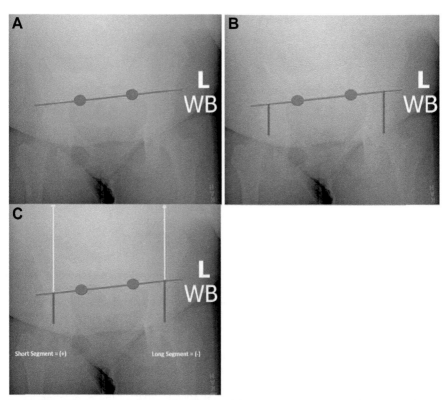

**Fig. 2.** *The ICLL Total LLD Method* is shown. (*A*) Demonstrating the right limb is shorter whereby a slope exists toward the shorter (right) limb. (*B*) The center of the femoral head is shown and a line is drawn to the pelvic line. (*C*) Total LLD = Short segment + Long Segment + Height of Blocks. Numeric measurements are gathered from the pelvic line to the top of the film or grid line (if available). Of note, all values that are for the longer limb will be negative and all values for the shorter limb will be designated as negative values.

femoral and tibial segments on the convex side along with a length measurement between the 2 using the central lateral femoral condyle to the lateral fibular neck. This value is then used to subtract the mechanical axis (from the center of the femoral head to the center of the ankle) to predict the specific amount of length to be achieved postcorrection (**Fig. 3**).

Contractures across joints are important to take into consideration as these may attribute to an apparent LLD, or may be compensation for a true LLD, as discussed later on in this article. Examples are hip adduction, knee flexion, and ankle plantarflexion. Hip adduction causes apparent shortening on the adducted side. Knee flexion contractures can also complicate a true limb length assessment. Methods have been developed to account for total limb length inequality in the setting of a sagittal plane contracture.[14] This involves the use of adjunctive lateral radiographic measurements. Ankle equinus may be primary or secondary.[15] Primary contracture is caused by pre-existing conditions such as spina bifida, cerebral palsy, or Charcot–Marie–Tooth. Unequal contracture between the 2 limbs may be confused with an apparent LLD. Secondary equinus is a reactive contracture to another event. In LLD, the patient may develop equinus on the shorter limb as compensation. Trauma, burns, and even

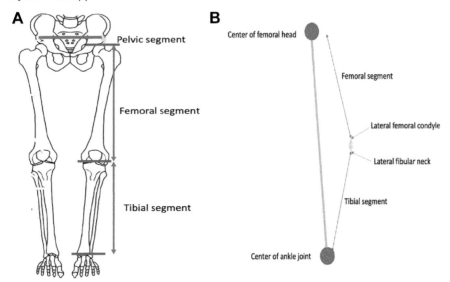

**Fig. 3.** ICLL individual segment assessment. (*A*) Diagrammatic representation without angular deformity presents outlining the pelvic, femoral, and tibial segments. (*B*) When deformity is present, length gain is determined by adding the femoral and tibial segments along with the convex measurement at the fibular neck and lateral condyle of the femur, followed by subtracting the mechanical axis on the concave side.

poliomyelitis can cause secondary equinus. Once again, the addition of lateral radiographs may be useful in properly measuring limb length in these patients.

Biomechanical compensation and gait adaptation allow for most to function with a limb length inequality. Literature accepts that 40% to 70% of the population has an unperceived LLD of about 2 cm. Inman reports that a normal center of gravity excursion is 5 cm vertical.[16] However, with the presence of LLD, this number can dramatically increase if compensation does not occur.[1] Many of these patterns are predictable and can be easily assessed. Most commonly, ankle equinus raises the foot whilst pelvis tilt lowers the pelvis to compensate on the shorter limb. In conjunction, an increase in knee flexion is often noted on the longer limb.

When evaluating a patient's gait, a reduction in stance time, stride length, and walking velocity are noticed on the shorter extremity. Cadence, on the other hand, is increased. Overtime these compensatory mechanisms can cause symptomatic muscle imbalances. Weakness of plantar flexors on the shorter extremity can affect equinus compensation during the stance phase of gait. A flexed knee posture on the longer extremity can lead to patellofemoral pathology and may not be tolerated. When this occurs, the quadriceps becomes weaker on the longer side; thereby, orienting the ground reaction force vector (GRV) posterior to the knee joint. Finally, the pelvis and spine compensate through hip abduction on the shorter side and adduction on the longer side. With prolonged compensation these joints become stiff and similar to the previous ankle compensation example, pelvic tilt may not occur and thus causing greater pain and discomfort to the patient. Similarly, if a patient has surgery for scoliosis deformity with a new fixed pelvic obliquity, this mechanism of compensation would no longer be available. The effects of LLD gait are reversible and have been demonstrated by Bhave and colleagues when the LLD is restored and equalized by limb lengthening reconstruction. In their study, preoperative reduced stance time and limited push-off were effectively restored after surgical intervention in a patient with a previous LLD of 4.6 mm.[17] (**Fig. 4**).

Prediction of LLD in the pediatric population historically had been based on prior data presented by Anderson and colleagues in 1964, which included length of the femur and tibia from age 1 to skeletal maturity across both sexes.[18] When an LLD is noted at birth, in the cases of congenital femoral deficiency, fibular hemimelia, tibial hemimelia, or hemiatrophy/hemihypertrophy, the short limb length could also be predicted based on observations of growth inhibition. Various equations/multipliers and ratios had been proposed in the literature to predict the length of the shorter extremity as well.[19,20] One approach in identifying short leg length at maturity was to multiply the ratio of the short leg length to the long leg length and the long leg length at skeletal maturity. Once the short leg at skeletal maturity was calculated, one would subtract this value from the predicted length of the long leg at skeletal maturity.[19,21]

In 1977, a straight line graph was created by Moseley in which Anderson's growth charts were implemented based on chronologic age.[22] Given the laborious nature of these calculations and given the fact that these charts cannot be used in an infant less than 1 year of age, more contemporary methods have been described factoring in both skeletal age and chronologic age. Paley and colleagues in 2000 developed the multiplier method and provide growth charts at every age from 0 to 16 as well as standard deviations and specific multipliers for boys and girls for both the tibia and the femur. Additionally, the multiplier method was found to be independent of race, nationality, and generation. Fortunately, this is currently available in text and through contemporary software for use on any mobile device.[4,5,23]

In pediatrics, there is a profound congenital influence in the diagnosis and management of limb length inequality. Essentially axial growth and unilateral discrepancy have been described as originating from either congenital, developmental, or acquired

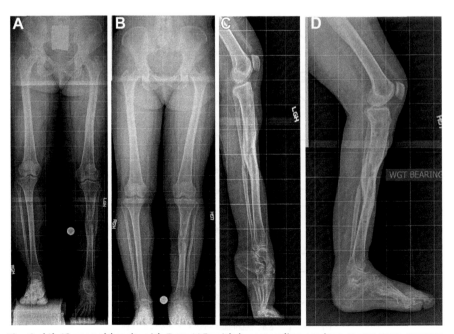

Fig. 4. (A) 48-year-old male with 7 cm LLD with longstanding equinus contracture compensation preoperative. (B) Postoperative weight-bearing erect long leg films demonstrating no further LLD. (C) Preoperative lateral foot/ankle/leg views. (D) Postoperative foot/ankle/leg views demonstrating the effects of gradual equinus correction.

etiologies. In 1982, Shapiro was able to delineate 5 different subtypes and demonstrate various potential differences of discrepancy with age progression.[24] (**Fig. 5**).

At times, postnatal LLD is observed in cases such as Ollier disease, Neurofibromatosis, Polio, and other factors leading to growth arrest. As one would expect, the rate of growth changes with age in accordance with normal growth parameters. Inhibition of the amount of growth remaining can also be calculated. This is accomplished by the ratio of growth of the short leg to the growth of the long leg. Two separate measurements of length are then taken. Inhibition is defined as the amount of interval growth of the short leg divided by the amount of interval growth of the long leg at a given time interval. Paley and colleagues recommend intervals of 6 to 12 months and radiographs must be taken after the growth disturbance.[1]

Malalignment and angular deformity may also predispose to LLD but is usually a result of congenital causes such as intrauterine dysplasia or hypoplasia of the epiphysis and not necessarily the physeal plate. In contrast to congenital angular deformity, congenital LLD is noted to be progressive and cease on physeal growth plate closure. Percentage of growth remaining for the distal femur, proximal tibia has been discussed in the literature with a determination that the distal femoral physis contributes 71% to the total growth of the femur and the proximal tibia contributes 57% to the total growth of the tibia.[25] Therefore, multiplying the femoral growth remaining of the femur by 0.71 and multiplying the tibial growth remaining by 0.57 can be used for accurate timing of epiphysiodesis if this is to be considered in the surgical management of LLD. According to some authors, the proportion of growth varies from 60% to 90% between the ages of 7 and 14 years for girls and 55% to 90% for boys (between the ages of 7 and 16 years old). Further, the growth contribution of the proximal tibia in girls varies from 50% to 80% at age 9 to 14 and in boys, varies from 50% to 80% for ages 10 to 16.[26] Following

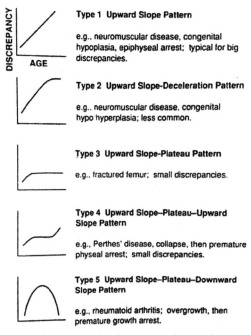

**Fig. 5.** Shapiro limb length discrepancy (LLD) types. As depicted, types 2 to 5 have an acceleration and deceleration component and therefore LLD can only be predicted in type 1. (*From* Shapiro F. Developmental patterns in lower-extremity length discrepancies. J Bone Joint Surg Am. 1982 Jun;64(5):639-51. PMID: 7085690.)

this work, Pritchett was able to further demonstrate the proximal and distal fibular contribution to growth at the physis. The group was able to determine in an evaluation of 123 boys and 121 girls 61% proximal and 39% distal growth contribution.[27] In keeping with these findings an investigation was performed by Karrholm which demonstrated the following consequences after ankle fracture: development of valgus compensation if the just the fibular growth plate was damaged, varus compensation, or neutral alignment after isolated tibial growth plate injury, and if fibular growth exceed proximal tibial growth a substantial growth arrest was noted (**Fig. 6**).[28]

## CONSERVATIVE MANAGEMENT

Conservative management can be considered when trying to accommodate for lesser length inequalities. If the patient is able to compensate for the length difference and is asymptomatic, then observation is an acceptable form of treatment. Some doctors may have the patient return yearly or every few years for re-evaluation of the LLD to make sure that it is not worsening through growth phases. For those who are symptomatic or have more obvious compensatory mechanisms that should be accommodated for, heel lifts either in shoes or in orthotics are the gold standard for conservative treatment. Heel lifts and built-up orthotics have been widely tolerated by children and adolescents more than adults. These can be low profile enough to be worn inside regular shoes. Unlike surgery which is far more definitive in treatment, lifts and orthotics can be adjusted as the pediatric patient continues to grow and develop. It is recommended that nonathletes will tolerate 0.75 inches of lift inside a shoe. Anything more than this, the patient may complain of a lack of space in the shoe or the feeling that their heel is not deep enough in the heel counter if they are wearing lower profile

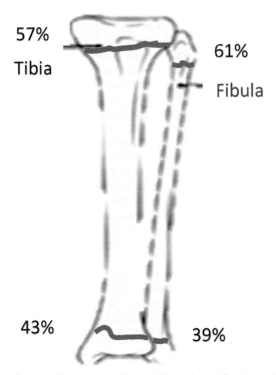

**Fig. 6.** Illustration of areas of proximal and distal physeal contribution to the growth of the tibia and fibula.

athletic shoes. Athletes are typically recommended 0.25 inches during sport. Less than 70% of military cadets in one study were willing to wear a heel lift up to 3 cm.[29] It is our experience that adding 2–3 mm per week assists in patient tolerance and comfort. If further length is desired, then custom shoes are a viable option. This allows for increased build-up externally at the sole of the shoe.

## SURGICAL MANAGEMENT

When a patient has greater than a 2 cm LLD and fails conservative treatment, surgical treatments may be considered. This can be addressed in several ways either by shortening the longer limb or by lengthening the shorter limb. During surgical planning, one not only should consider the etiology of the LLD but also the social factors that each patient presents with. Age, activity demands, as well as patient and parent's ability to comply, are very important when determining which procedure is best suited for the patient.

Epiphysiodesis is indicated when there is a limb length inequality of 2–5 cm. It involves altering or stopping bone growth at the physis in a developing child. This is performed on the longer limb and allows the shorter limb to remain untouched and continue growing to catch up in length. The procedure was first described by Phemister in 1938. It has since evolved in technique.[30] In standard practice, the peripheral margins of the medial and lateral physis are ablated, commonly by the use of drilling. Other techniques have cited the use of staples to compress the physis. This stunts growth but is theoretically reversible once the staples have been removed, as no actual ablation occurred within the physis itself. Although any physis can be used, the most common is the physes about the knee. Green noted slower rates of growth per year by approximately 27% for the proximal tibia, 38% for the distal femur, and 65% for combined epiphysiodesis of both plates.[31] This is a much larger proportion of growth arrest than other locations in the lower extremity. By performing an epiphysiodesis on only one side of the growth plate—or hemiepiphysiodesis—one can also compensate for any angular discrepancies. For example, a lateral hemiepiphysiodesis will arrest the lateral side of the growth plate. The medial side will continue to grow, thus persuading a valgus attitude. To treat a varus ankle, lateral hemiepiphysiodesis should be performed. To treat a valgus ankle, a medial hemiepiphysiodesis should be performed.

Epiphysiodesis tends to be favored in pediatric patients as it is far less involved than other limb length surgeries. The incisions and structural results are often cosmetically more appealing. Patients are able to maintain their activity level with much shorter recovery times following surgery. Epiphysiodesis also tends to be less expensive than lengthening procedures. The biggest pitfall to this surgery is that it can be somewhat unpredictable. Although Mosley's graphs and Anderson's growth charts can help us predict when growth plates may close in adolescents, it does not account for growth on an individual level. For individuals, some may have grown more rapidly earlier or later than anticipated. Incorrect timing of surgery may result in a less than perfect result following an epiphysiodesis. It is also important to remember that this surgery is compensatory and not corrective.

Corrective procedures often involve osteotomies and subsequent lengthening of the shortened limb. This can be performed acutely or gradually. Gradual lengthening, or distraction osteogenesis, is often preferred as it allows for more lengthening over long periods of time. Gaining too much length too quickly can stretch out neurovascular structures and cause injury. The patient is also at an increased risk of delayed or nonunion with acute lengthening.

Instead, gradual lengthening has fallen into favor. It involves (1) a low-energy periosteum sparing osteotomy and (2) subsequent slow progressive distraction of the bone ends. Lengthening can be done over an intramedullary nail, an external fixator, or a combination of both. Before committing to any lengthening procedures, it is important to assess the patient's psychological status, social status, and outcome expectations. These procedures often require many months of compliance and activity modification to achieve a desired length and outcome. Especially when operating on a pediatric patient, it is also imperative to have the parents fully informed as well.

As noted earlier in this article, radiographic studies to assess length needed and any angular deformities associated with an LLD are first required. Today, software-based deformity analysis from a CT is preferred as this can compute length, angulation, rotation, and the CORA of the deformity.

The first step in distraction osteogenesis is performing the osteotomy. Good technique to form good osseous callus prevents thermal damage, uses careful bone separation, creates vascular bone surfaces, respects the periosteal sleeve, and gradually pulls the bony segments apart overtime.[32] Gigli saw, oscillating saw, and osteotomes have all been used to perform osteotomies. When possible, a corticotomy should be performed instead of an osteotomy. This separates the cortex only, preserving both the medullary canal and the periosteum to maintain the maximum blood supply to the bone. Although the osteotomy or corticotomy can be performed at various locations along a long bone, the metaphyseal diaphyseal junction is ideal as there is the extensive blood supply to this area. Other considerations for location include the CORA of the deformity, having adequate fixation above and below the osteotomy, and interruption of surrounding structures such as muscular attachments.

After the osteotomy is performed, it must be fixated. Monorail external fixators are less cumbersome than ring fixators, but are only indicated in singular plain deformities. More commonly, ring fixators are applied. This allows for increased stability and multiplanar correction. Taylor spatial frames (TSFs) have gained popularity over the years. These use a computer-generated sequence in deformity correction. This tells the patient or his or her parents how and when to adjust each individually labeled strut. Therefore, adjusting and lengthening are far less confusing for the patient and a more precise correction can be achieved. Unfortunately, these TSFs come at a significantly higher price than regular ring fixators. The pitfall of any external fixation is that it is significantly bulkier and requires more attentive care. 96% of patients will develop some form of pin site infection.[33] This rate has even been shown to be higher than this the longer the external fixator remains on. Iizarov's technique suggests a 7-day latency phase following the osteotomy. The second phase is the distraction phase in which bone is lengthened at a rate of 1 mm/d performed in 4 increments of 0.25 mm for improved tolerance.[34] Once the desired length is achieved, the frame should remain on for twice as long as it took to achieve the length. This is considered the consolidation phase which allows new bone to mature. Complying with this technique leads to long periods in an external fixator. For example, if a patient needs 5 cm in length, then the external fixator should remain on for over 3.5 months.

Lengthening over nail (LON) aims to reduce the complications that are inevitable when in external fixation for too long. The concept was first introduced by Bost and Larson in 1956. An intramedullary nail is inserted at the time of osteotomy. The osteotomy is still lengthened over time through an external fixator but once the desired length is achieved, then the nail is locked and the external fixator can be removed. This reduces the risk of increased pin site infections and loosening of wire. The nail holds the position while the distracted site continues to ossify. With the same principles applied, percutaneous plating has also been explored as a viable option for lengthening and fixation instead of a nail.[35]

With the advancement of technology, nails have been developed to have lengthening capabilities. The self-lengthening IMNs are considered for those with solely a limb length deformity (without rotational or angulation components) and have made it possible to eliminate the need for external fixation. This allows the patient to have a higher activity level while lengthening, fewer scars, no risk for pin site infections, and better psychological well-being. Although the first lengthening nail was implanted in the 1970s, newer techniques have been far more successful and reproducible.

The intramedullary skeletal kinematic nail (ISKN) designed by Orthofix (Lewisville, Tx) is made for humerus, femur, and tibial lengthening. It uses a ratchet mechanism that, when the patient is ambulating, takes the physiologic 3 to 9° of internal rotation and converts this into the distraction of the nail. One potential problem with this technique is that it does depend on the activity level of the patient, inactive patients may require additional lengthening under general anesthesia if they are not able to maintain the required rate of distraction through activity. Lengthening of the nail is also irreversible. The patient is given an external magnetic reader to make sure that they are not over lengthening too quickly. Overall, the ISKN allows for 50 to 80 mm of distraction.

The Precice and Precice 2 nails from Ellipse Technologies (Irvine, Ca) and now Nuvasive (San Diego, Ca) are an example of magnetically controlled lengthening nails. External remote control is held over the magnetic mechanism to trigger lengthening within the nail. It is the only nail that also has a reverse mechanism if the nail is accidentally over lengthened. It allows for up to 8 cm in the femur and 6.5 cm in the tibia. The femoral nail can be inserted either antegrade or retrograde. In a study by Iliadis, 50 consecutive limbs were lengthened using the Precice systems. The mean age at surgery was 15 years old (12–17). Their mean preoperative length discrepancy was 49 mm (20–90) with a mean achieved lengthening of 46.5 mm (20–80). Overall, they found that their nail accuracy was 96% with a reliability of 90%.[36] Newer research continues to be published showing promising results for these less invasive, advanced lengthening techniques.

## DISCUSSION

The body's inability to compensate leads to pain and persistent deformity. A limb length inequality can ultimately change the strength of various muscles involved in compensation and lead to abnormal excursion of the center of gravity. This can affect the entire kinetic chain with gait, leading to higher metabolic demands and earlier arthritic changes at joints. Although long-term consequences of LLD are fortunately not evident in the pediatric population, it is imperative to be able to recognize this pathology, particularly in the pediatric population to prevent the harmful long-term sequelae.

Limb length can be evaluated both clinically and radiographically. Radiographic assessment is preferred over clinical assessment alone and has implications both for surgical and conservative management. Weight Bearing lower extremity x-rays can be a useful tool for in-office evaluation of LLD. More specifically, total lower extremity CTs can be run through new computer software to precisely determine LLF, angulation, and rotational deformities.

These allow for more precise surgical planning. The TSFs allow for accurate, user friendly directions on daily frame adjustments following surgery. Newer intramedullary nails also use the information gained through CTs to compute precise lengthening. Although Ilizarov's principles of distraction osteogenesis pioneered the world of deformity correction, these newer technologies have allowed patients to maintain activity while lengthening and decreased the risk of pin site infections. One can expect continued advances in computer-guided, custom lengthening techniques in the future.

## CLINICS CARE POINTS

- Clinical evaluation of lower limb discrepancy has been demonstrated to be accurate and reproducible through the use of modern digital imaging assessment.
- When apparent limb length inequality is suspected it is important to measure segmental differences in femoral, tibial, and foot height as to not over-estimate LLD.
- Conservative management for less than 2cm of LLD is reasonable.
- Epiphysiodesis surgery has been revolutionized through the use of smart phone and tablet applications which can aid the surgeon in timing their procedure by analyzing growth remaining at the affected extremity.
- Distraction osteogenesis remains the mainstay of regenerate bone formation with recent advancement made through the use of computer-assisted hexapod external fixation and magnetized intramedullary nailing; thereby, avoiding issues with pin site infection and reducing the time required for immobilization within an external fixator device.
- It is important to be mindful of secondary joint contractures that can occur after surgical reconstruction.

## DISCLOSURES

Jacob Wynes – Consultant Smith and Nephew.

## REFERENCES

1. Paley D. Principles of deformity correction. In: Corr. 3rd printing. Rev edition. 1st edition. Berlin: Springer-Verlag; 2005.
2. Anderson M, Messner MB, Green WT. Distribution of lengths of the normal femur and tibia in children from one to eighteen years of age. J Bone Joint Surg Am 1964;46:1197–202.
3. Aldegheri R, Agostini S. A chart of anthropometric values. J Bone Joint Surg Br 1993;75(1):86–8.
4. Herzenberg JE, Bhave A, Standard SC. Multiplier App. Version 7.0. Available at: https://www.limblength.org/about-us/physician-education/multiplier-mobile-app/.
5. Paley D. Paley growth. Version 3.0. Available at: https://apps.apple.com/us/app/paley-growth/id435195238.
6. Gurney B. Leg length discrepancy. Gait Posture 2002;15(2):195–206.
7. Khamis S, Carmeli E. A new concept for measuring leg length discrepancy. J Orthop 2017;14(2):276–80.
8. Brady RJ, Dean JB, Skinner TM, et al. Limb length inequality: clinical implications for assessment and intervention. J Orthop Sports Phys Ther 2003;33(5):221–34.
9. Gross MT, Burns CB, Chapman SW, et al. Reliability and validity of rigid lift and pelvic leveling device method in assessing functional leg length inequality. J Orthop Sports Phys Ther 1998;27(4):285–94.
10. Bell JS, Thompson WA. Modified spot scanography. Am J Roentgenol Radium Ther 1950;63(6):915–6.
11. Green WT, Wyatt GM, Anderson M. Orthoroentgenography as a method of measuring the bones of the lower extremities. J Bone Joint Surg Am 1946; 28:60–5.
12. Tachdijian MO. Pediatric orthopedics. Philadelphia: W.B. Saunders; 1972.
13. Tokarowski A, Piechota L, Wojciechowski P, et al. Pomiar długości kończyn dolnych przy uzyciu tomografu komputerowego [Measurement of lower extremity

length using computed tomography]. Chir Narzadow Ruchu Ortop Pol 1995; 60(2):123–7.

14. Amstutz HC, Sakai DN. Equalization of leg length. Clin Orthop Relat Res 1978; 136:2–6.

15. Gourdine-Shaw MC, Lamm BM, Herzenberg JE, et al. Equinus deformity in the pediatric patient: causes, evaluation, and management. Clin Podiatr Med Surg 2010;27(1):25–42.

16. Inman VT, Ralston HJ, Todd F. Human locomotion. In: Rose J, Gamble JG, editors. Human walking. Baltimore: Williams & Wilkins; 1994. p. 1–22.

17. Bhave A, Paley D, Herzenberg JE. Improvement in gait parameters after lengthening for the treatment of limb-length discrepancy. J Bone Joint Surg Am 1999; 81(4):529–34.

18. Anderson M, Green WT. Lengths of the femur and the tibia: Norms derived from orthoroentgenograms of children from five years of age until epiphyseal closure. Am J Dis Child 1948;75:279–90.

19. Asmutz HC. National history and treatment of congenital absence of the fibula. J Bone Joint Surg Am 1969;54:1349.

20. Pappas AM. Congenital abnormalities of the femur and related lower extremity malformations: classification and treatment. J Pediatr Orthop 1983;3:45–60.

21. Hootnick D, Boyd NA, Fixsen JA, et al. The natural history and management of congenital short tibia with dysplasia or absence of the fibula. J Bone Joint Surg Br 1977;59:267–71.

22. Moseley CF. A Straight-line graph for leg-length discrepancies. J Bone Joint Surg Am 1978;59:174–9.

23. Paley D, Bhave A, Herzenberg JE, et al. Multiplier method for predicting limb-length discrepancy. J Bone Joint Surg Am 2000;82(10):1432–46.

24. Shapiro F. Developmental patterns in lower-extremity length discrepancies. J Bone Joint Surg Am 1982;64:639–51.

25. Anderson M, Green WT, Messner MB. Growth and predictions of growth in the lower extremities. J Bone Joint Surg Am 1963;45:1–14.

26. Pritchett JW. Longitudinal growth and growth-plate activity in the lower extremity. Clin Orthop Relat Res 1992;275:274–9.

27. Pritchett JW. Growth and growth prediction of the fibula. Clin Orthop Relat Res 1997; 334:251–6.

28. Kärrholm J, Hansson LI, Selvik G. Changes in tibiofibular relationships due to growth disturbances after ankle fractures in children. J Bone Joint Surg Am 1984;66(8):1198–210.

29. Goss DL, Moore JH. Compliance wearing a heel lift during 8 weeks of military training in cadets with limb length inequality. J Orthop Sports Phys Ther 2004; 34(3):126–31.

30. Phemister DB. Epiphysiodèse pour l'égalisation de la longueur des membres inférieurs et la correction d'autres difformités du squelette [Epiphysiodesis for equalizing the length of the lower extremities and for correcting other deformities of the skeleton]. Mem Acad Chir (Paris) 1950;76(26–27):758–63.

31. Green W, Anderson M. Experiences with epiphyseal arrest in correcting discrepancies in length of the lower extremities in infantile paralysis. J Bone Joint Surg 1947;29:659–75.

32. Aldegheri R. Femoral callotasis. J Pediatr Orthop B 1997;6:42–7.

33. Antoci V, Ono CM, Antoci V Jr, et al. Pin-tract infection during limb lengthening using external fixation. Am J Orthop (Belle Mead NJ) 2008;37:E150–4.

34. Ilizarov GA. The Tension-stress effect on the genesis and growth of tissues. Part I. The influence of stability of fixation and soft-tissue preservation. Clin Orthop Relat Res 1989;238:249–81.

35. Kulkarni R, Singh N, Kulkarni GS, et al. Limb lengthening over plate. Indian J Orthop 2012;46(3):339–45.

36. Iliadis AD, Palloni V, Wright J, et al. Pediatric lower limb lengthening using the PRECICE nail: our experience with 50 cases. J Pediatr Orthop 2021;41(1):e44–9.

# Tarsal Coalitions

Gan Golshteyn, MS, DPM[a],*, Harry P. Schneider, DPM[b]

## KEYWORDS

- Pediatrics • Foot and ankle • Tarsal coalition • Tarsal coalition resection
- Foot and ankle surgery • Foot and ankle pain • Flatfeet • Tarsal coalition radiology

## KEY POINTS

- Tarsal coalition is a relatively common congenital foot and ankle condition caused by failure of mesenchymal segmentation leading to abnormal boney growth.
- The most common tarsal coalitions are talocalcaneal coalitions and calcaneonavicular coalitions.
- Conservative treatment consists of immobilization, NSAIDs, and casting for symptomatic patients.
- Surgical treatment for symptomatic tarsal coalition consists of resection and/or arthrodesis.

## INTRODUCTION

Tarsal coalitions are recognized as a congenital anomaly whereby the two or more bones of the hindfoot and midfoot are fused resulting in limitation of foot motion and pain. While the etiology of tarsal coalition is unknown, it is characterized as an unifactorial autosomal dominant pattern of inheritance with variable penetrance and roughly 50% bilaterality.[1–3] It has been reported that tarsal coalition affect approximately 1% to 2% of the general population, and about 25% of patients become symptomatic.[3–5] Subsequently, tarsal coalitions were found to be the cause of painful flatfeet in adolescents and young adults.[6,7] Calcaneonavicular coalitions where first anatomically described by Cruveilheir in 1829, and the first radiographic presentation of a tarsal coalition was written by Kirmisson in 1898, roughly 3 years after Roentgen's discovery of X-rays.[8–11] Slomann, in 1921, demonstrated 5 cases of calcaneonavicular coalition on an oblique foot radiograph, and in 1927, Bagley resected a calcaneonavicular coalition and noted that the coalition was associated with peroneal spastic flatfoot.[10,12–14]

In 1877, Zuckerlandl anatomically identified a talocalcaneal coalition, and in 1934, Korvin used axial radiograph imaging of the calcaneus to clearly identify a talocalcaneal coalition.[15,16] Harris and Beath, in 1948, popularized the radiograph examination

[a] The Pediatric Orthopedic Center, Cedar Knolls, NJ, USA; [b] Department of Surgery, Cambridge Health Alliance, Harvard Medical School, 1493 Cambridge Street, Cambridge, MA 02139, USA
* Corresponding author. 6145 North Thesta Street, Fresno, CA 93710.
*E-mail address:* gan.golshteyn@gmail.com

Clin Podiatr Med Surg 39 (2022) 129–142
https://doi.org/10.1016/j.cpm.2021.08.004
0891-8422/22/© 2021 Elsevier Inc. All rights reserved.

of Korvin's calcaneal axial view to show that talocalcaneal coalitions are a cause of peroneal spastic flatfoot. Harris and Beath demonstrated the bridging of the middle facet of the subtalar joint as a descriptive factor of talocalcaneal coalitions.[4,7,8] Although talocalcaneal and calcaneonavicular tarsal coalitions are the most commonly identified pathologies, other tarsal coalitions have been noted in literature. Developing a clinical understanding of tarsal coalitions as well as developing a step-wise conservative and surgical approach for their treatment can alleviate patient symptomatology and provide excellent long-term benefits.

## ETIOLOGY

Although the etiology of tarsal coalition is unknown, the most likely cause is failure of normal segmentation of the fetal tarsal during development. In 1896, Pfitzner studied the anatomy of 524 feet and suggested that accessory ossicles were incorporated into the adjacent normal tarsal bones as he observed sesamoid bones and accessory os-sicles at the anatomic areas where coalitions had occurred (**Fig. 1**).[17] In his study, he noted 2 of the 524 feet autopsied had an incidence of coalition, 0.38%. Leboucq, Sol-ger, and other authors believed the cause of tarsal coalition was a failure of segmen-tation of primitive mesenchyme.[18,19] Currently, the most widely accepted theory of the etiology of tarsal coalition is the one by Harris and Beath in 1948 and Harris in 1955. They examined 3619 army recruits and found a tarsal coalition incidence of 1 of 3619 (.03%), making note that tarsal coalition is due to failure of segmentation and differen-tiation in embryos.[6,20,21] In 1974, Leonard examined the hereditary transmission of tarsal coalition.[1] He evaluated the first-degree relatives (parents and siblings) of 31 pa-tients with tarsal coalition. Of these, 98 first-degree relatives (39%) had tarsal coali-tions demonstrated by radiographs. He concluded that tarsal coalition is an unifactorial disorder of autosomal dominant inheritance, with nearly full pene-trance.[1,22] Other reported cases of familial occurrence of coalitions have been cited in literature. Boyd in 1944 described a family with bilateral talonavicular bars in three generations.[22] Wray and Herndon described calcaneonavicular coalitions in three

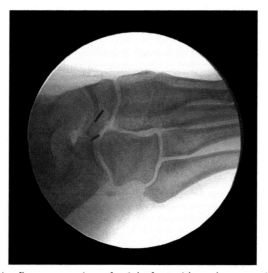

**Fig. 1.** Intraoperative fluoroscopy view of a right foot with a calcaneonavicular coalition us-ing 2 × 0.062-inch K wires as a guide for the osteotomy.

generations of a family and proposed that this phenomenon represented an auto-somal dominant inheritance with reduced penetrance.[23] Calcaneonavicular bars and talocalcaneal bridges are the 2 most common types of tarsal coalitions, accounting for nearly 90% of all coalitions, with clinical presentation between the ages of 10 to 12 and 12 to 16 years, respectively.[24,25]

## CLINICAL FINDINGS

Tarsal coalitions are an unusual cause of foot symptoms that are commonly misdiag-nosed or excessively sought after. A patient with a tarsal coalition may be devoid of symp-toms, and an incidental finding on routine plain film radiograph may lead to the diagnosis. Although tarsal coalitions occur in less than 1% of the population, many patients are asymptomatic, while others develop pain, recurrent ankle sprains, muscle spasms, and limitation of joint motion, as well as a possible pes planus deformity on clinical exam-ination.[2,26] Jack noted that 5 of 23 patients (22%) had no symptoms within 30 cases of peroneal spastic flatfoot.[27,28] Many theories have been discussed surrounding the origin of peroneal spasm and whether or not a tarsal coalition predisposes the patient to devel-oping other clinical symptoms, such as anterior tibial spasm with a varus deformity.[29–31] Rarely is a tarsal coalition associated with a cavus foot type.[29–32] A thorough understand-ing of the common clinical findings associated with tarsal coalitions in the pediatric pop-ulation allows for appropriate management and prevention of future pathologies.

Peroneal spasm occurs from a biomechanical "splinting" of the subtalar joint, thereby reducing the pressure of the subtalar joint.[33] This results in secondary adap-tive shortening of the peroneal muscle in response to heel valgus.[32] Electromyography studies have shown spasticity of the peroneus longus muscle in patients with a coa-lition, as well as the soleus and gastrocnemius muscles.[32,34,35] The "triad" of peroneal spastic pes planovalgus has been reported as spasms of the peroneal muscles, pain-ful pes planovalgus deformity, and a tarsal coalition.[33,34]

Initially, the patient will complain of a deep and aching painful area that is associated with the tarsal coalition. The patient may be able to localize the pain to the dorsum and/or dorsal-lateral aspect of the midfoot, anterolateral ankle, or the sinus tarsi upon palpation. The onset of pain is usually insidious, usually developing after an acute injury, such as ankle sprain, or after some unusual activity, such as excessive walking or running.[36] Conway and cowell noted that symptoms associated with tarsal coalitions appear in the second decade of life, and it is most likely related to the ossi-fication of the fibrous or cartilaginous coalition.[37] A similar notion is agreed upon by many researchers as they have stated that all coalitions are initially cartilaginous, and as they ossify upon aging, the patient may then begin to experience pain in the coalition site. Cowell states that talonavicular coalitions ossify from ages 3 to 5 years, calcaneonavicular coalition ossifies from ages 8 to 12 years, and a talocalcaneal coa-lition ossifies from ages 12 to 16 years.[36,38–40]

The clinical presentation and findings of a talocalcaneal coalition are commonly described as decreased subtalar joint motion and midtarsal joint motion, alongside a pes planovalgus deformity.[32,37] In addition, the patient may indicate that the pain en-compasses the entire rearfoot.[36,38] Limitation with subtalar joint inversion is a clinical finding and may be associated with peroneal spasm.[38] If an incomplete coalition is present, as ossification progresses, range of motion at the subtalar joint and midtarsal joint will decrease, resulting in pain, increase in onset of ankle sprains, and sports in-juries.[38,41] Owing to the absence of inflammatory cells that have been reported in his-topathological studies, it is believed that pain associated with tarsal coalitions is secondary to mechanical stress from the periosteum surrounding the ossifying coalition.[42–44] Cass and Camasta noted that on clinical examination, patients may exhibit mild to deep pain within the subtalar joint with passive range of motion.[32] During open kinetic chain examination, a patient may have a valgus position of the rearfoot, as well as an equinus position at the level of the ankle, loss of medial longitudinal arch height, and forefoot protonation. If the coalition is unilateral, such characteristics are identifiably relative to the contralateral limb.[32,42]

## RADIOGRAPHIC EVALUATION

Diagnosing tarsal coalitions begins with plain film radiographs, in the form of weight-bearing anteroposterior, oblique, and lateral images. Radiographs are examined for distortion of normal bone architecture suggesting union (fibrous or bony) between the involved bones.[45] Beaking of the talus can be visualized on lateral plain film radiographs. A talocalcaneal coalition can be visualized on lateral plain film radiographs as narrowing on the posterior subtalar joint, rounding of the lateral talar process, obliteration of the middle subtalar joint facet, and/or flattening/concavity of the talar neck.[45] The classic C-sign, originally described by Brown and colleagues, is visualized on lateral plain film radiographs as a bean-shaped density due to the prominent inferior outline of the sustentaculum tali to create an overlap or a hyperdense region in combination with the medial outline of the talar dome and a bony bridge between the talar down and the sustentaculum tali.[45,46] Talar beaking refers to a flaring/osseus hypertrophy of the superior dorsal aspect of the talar head, secondary to an aberrant hinge-like motion of the navicular upon the talus with dorsiflexion seen in patients with a tarsal coalition.[45,47,48] A calcaneonavicular coalition becomes apparent on the 45-degree lateral oblique radiograph as either a complete osseous union or extension of the anterior neck of the calcaneus to the navicular, recognized as the anteater nose sign.[45,47–49]

The Harris calcaneal axial view is a critical radiographic view used to detect tarsal coalitions.[4] In a normal hindfoot, without the presence of a tarsal coalition, the posterior and middle facet are in parallel planes, approximately 45° to the sole of the foot, and the middle facet is perpendicular to the axis of the tibia.[50] Angle of the middle facet greater than 20° off horizontal axis is consistent with a coalition, even if the joint space is open (Wheeless Text Book).

Advanced imaging modalities play an imperative role in the evaluation and diagnosing of a tarsal coalition. Crim and Kjeldsberg performed a two-phased study in 150 patients with a mean age of 29 years in reviewing tarsal coalition using plain film radiographs.[51] The authors noted that plain film radiographs are 100% sensitive and 88% specific to diagnosing talocalcaneal coalitions and 80% sensitive and 97% specific to diagnosing calcaneonavicular coalitions.[51] Computed tomography (CT) has superseded plain film radiography in diagnostic accuracy of tarsal coalitions, alongside its added benefit of detecting early degenerative joint disease at adjacent surfaces.[45] In the pediatric population, MRI is used because of less radiation exposure and its ability to detect fibrous coalitions. Emery and colleagues reviewed 40 MRI and CT scans taken on 20 patients with symptomatic tarsal coalitions.[52] The authors determined that CT scanning was 94% sensitive and 100% specific, whereas MRI was 88% sensitive and 100% specific; 71% of patients had a fibrous coalition.[45,52,53] Therefore, the study of choice depends on the patient age, cost-effectiveness, additional pathologies, and clinical findings.

## CLASSIFICATION

Tarsal coalitions were historically classified according to (1) etiologic type, (2) anatomic type, and (3) tissue type.[54] Tarsal coalitions can be classified according to their etiology: either congenital or acquired.[54,55] Acquired coalitions are less common than congenital and may result from arthritis, trauma, neoplasms, infection, or other predisposing factors. The causes of acquired tarsal coalitions can lead to varying degrees of joint stiffness with and without complete restriction of motion. In consideration to all age groups, acquired tarsal coalitions are a frequent cause of symptomatic peroneal spastic flatfoot.[36,55,56] Congenital tarsal coalitions remain the most frequently reported tarsal coalitions, although the etiology remains unknown. However, it is important to note that classifying tarsal coalitions by etiology does not generally ascertain the best possible treatment plan.[54] Tachdijian in 1985 created a classification system that subdivides coalitions into bones that are abnormally united or part of a complex malformation (**Fig. 2**).[8,56] Tachdjian's classification suggests the importance of examining and assessing the entirety of the foot and ankle complex when an apparently local or isolated coalition is identified.[8,56] The third type of classifying tarsal coalitions is based on tissue type of their union. This classification helps describe the coalition, which may be a synostosis (osseous union), a synchondrosis (a cartilaginous union), and/or a syndesmosis (fibrous union). A synostosis may further be subdivided into a complete coalition, in which all joint motions are relatively absent, or an incomplete coalition, which is a fibrocartilaginous coalition with varying amounts of interposed cartilaginous or fibrous tissue, therefore, allowing some joint motion.[8] It is important to note that such classification systems, even when combined, only provide descriptive characteristics of tarsal coalitions and fail to establish a surgical treatment plan.

Given this deficiency within the classification system of tarsal coalitions, Downey proposed the Articular Classification System as a surgical classification system for tarsal coalitions.[38] The classification system is based on the articular relationship of the bones involved in the coalition and the indirect effect that the coalition may have on surrounding joints of the foot and ankle. The classification system is not meant to be all inclusive but considers several important factors, such as patients age, relationship of the bones forming the coalition (articular involvement), and the degree of secondary arthritics changes within the foot and ankle, in the development of a surgical treatment plan. **Fig. 3** introduces the classification system by distinguishing between juveniles (osseous immaturity) and adults (osseous maturity).[38,56] The level of osseous maturity is further divided into extra-articular coalitions and intra-articular

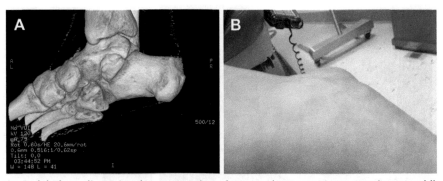

**Fig. 2.** (A) Three-dimensional reconstruction of CT scan demonstrating a prominent meddle facet. (B) Clinical photo of the "double medial malleolus" defined by Rocchi (A). Note the hypertrophied medial face as it is related to a bony overgrowth relative to normal, therefore, giving the appearance of a double bony prominence noted inferior to medial malleolus.

coalitions. Extra-articular coalitions are recognized as tarsal coalitions that occur outside a normal joint, commonly referred to as bars. Stormont and colleagues recognized that calcaneonavicular coalition bars were found to be the most common type, followed by talocalcaneal coalition bridges, which are intra-articular coalitions. Intra-articular coalitions occur at normal joint sites and are commonly known as bridges **(Fig. 4)**.[36,38] The classification system is further subdivided into the presence or absence of secondary arthritic changes to the surrounding joints. The Articular Classification System is not meant to be all-inclusive, and it does describe important considerations used in the development of any treatment regimen.[8] In addition to the factors Downey described in his original classification, he recently recommended that the size of the coalition and the degree of heel valgus should also be considered in the treatment plan.[36,38]

## CONSERVATIVE TREATMENT

Conservative treatment of tarsal coalitions has been shown in the literature to be successful in the short to medium term.[57,58] The long-term concern is always compensation at surrounding joints due to abnormal valgus alignment and decreased range of motion. Conservative treatment consists of University of California at Berkeley Laboratory (UCBL)-type orthotics to help decrease the range of motion of the area. Similarly, a supramalleolar orthotic or ankle brace that limits rear foot ankle range of motion will also alleviate symptoms. Physical therapy has been shown to help by building up the collateral muscle strength.[57]

## SURGICAL TREATMENT

The preferred surgical treatment for calcaneonavicular bar is resection because it is an extra-articular coalition. The incision is curvilinear and extends from the tip of the fibula extending over the sinus tarsi to the level of the fourth metatarsal cuboid joint. The extensor digitorum brevis muscle is reflected superiorly, and the peroneal tendons are reflected inferiorly. Anatomic landmarks include the calcaneocuboid joint and the sinus tarsi. The dissection is then continued medially to the lateral aspect of the talonavicular joint. This easily exposes the calcaneonavicular bar. It is very important

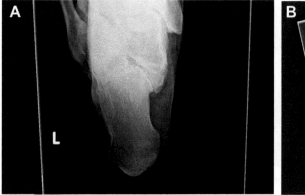
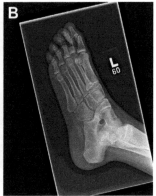

**Fig. 3.** (*A*) Calcaneal axial view of the left hindfoot demonstrating a middle facet coalition of the talocalcaneal joint. (*B*) Medial oblique view of the left foot demonstrating a calcaneonavicular coalition.

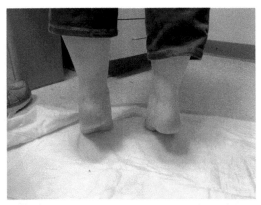

**Fig. 4.** Clinical examination of an adult patient with lack of resupination of the right rear-foot secondary to tarsal coalition.

to understand the anatomy of this area. One must protect the calcaneocuboid joint and the lateral aspect of the talar head. It is also important to resect a rectangular wedge of bone rather than a trapezoidal or triangular piece which is a common mistake. The senior author uses two 0.062-inch K wires as a guide for the osteotomy (see **Fig. 1**). The K wire runs obliquely from dorsal lateral to plantar medial and will exit into the medial longitudinal arch (**Fig. 5**). One should be able to insert the thumb in between the calcaneus and the navicular once the bone has been fully resected. Failure to fully resect the bone and/or leaving a narrower gap plantarly will lead to recurrence (**Fig. 6**). **Fig. 7**A and B shows a calcaneonavicular coalition that recurred in 2 years after inadequate plantar resection (see **Fig. 7**A, B).

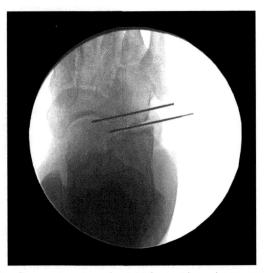

**Fig. 5.** Intraoperative fluoroscopy view of a right foot with a calcaneonavicular coalition using 2 × 0.062-inch K wires that run obliquely from the dorsal lateral to plantar medial and will exit into the medial longitudinal arch.

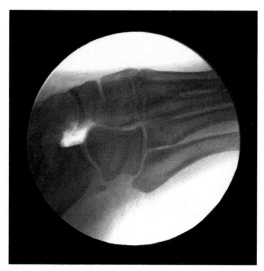

**Fig. 6.** Intraoperative fluoroscopy view of a right foot after a calcaneonavicular coalition. Notice the complete resection of the coalition site with no boney apposition as noted in **Fig. 5**.

Once the bone has been resected from the calcaneonavicular bar, it was originally described to insert the extensor digitorum brevis muscle belly into the space that the coalition originally occupied. However, there were still some recurrences as the muscle belly did not extend all the way plantarly. The original idea of a suture button has

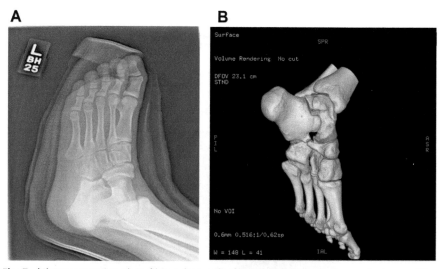

**Fig. 7.** (*A*) Postoperative plain film radiograph obtained after a calcaneonavicular coalition resection. Note the inadequate resection of the coalition site with minor joint space noted. (*B*) Three-dimensional reconstruction of CT scan of the left foot. Demonstrating the regrowth of the inferior portion of the previously inadequately resected calcaneonavicular coalition.

fallen out of favor. Additionally, some patients did not like the cosmetic appearance of missing tissue from the dorsolateral foot. More recently, other spacers have been used. Examples of spacers include fat graft, collagen graft, amniotic tissue, or bone wax. These all have the advantage of retaining the normal anatomy of the extensor digitorum muscle belly and allow for appropriate filling of the resection space (**Fig. 8**).

Resection of a talocalcaneal middle facet coalition can be performed by resectional arthroplasty versus arthrodesis. If the patient has a double medial malleolus, then it is quite easy to understand the location of the middle facet coalition. If not, making an incision on the medial aspect of the foot and understanding the coalition location can be quite daunting. Once the incision is carried down to bone, it can be difficult to understand where the talus ends in the calcaneus begins. Therefore, the senior author inserts a 0.062-inch K wire across the sinus tarsi and then penetrates the coalition on the medial side (**Fig. 9**). The K wire is inserted until the skin on the

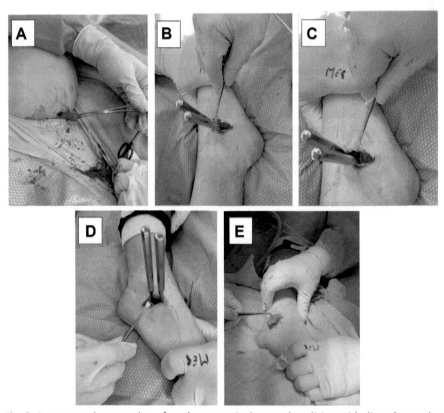

**Fig. 8.** Intraoperative resection of a calcaneonavicular tarsal coalition with direct harvesting of fat graft from the buttock in an 11-year-old patient. (*A*) The direct harvesting of the fat graft from the buttock before tarsal coalition resection. (*B*) Two parallel osteotomes are directed at the anterior process of the calcaneus and the lateral border of the navicular at the area of coalition with direct visualization and fluoroscopy. (*C, D*) The angle of the osteotomes and visualization of the calcaneonavicular coalition. (*E*) After resection of the coalition, direct implantation of the fat graft that was previously harvested from the buttock and soaked in sterile saline.

medial aspect of the foot is tented. This gives the exact location of the tarsal coalition (**Fig. 10**). The K wire is then removed. A 4-cm incision is then made over the area identified by the K wire. The posterior tibial tendon is reflected superiorly, and the flexor digitorum longus tendon is reflected inferiorly. One will see the location where the K wire penetrated the bone at the area of the middle facet coalition. Resection can be performed with a saw, osteotome, arthroscope, or rongeur. It is important to resect enough to allow range of motion of the subtalar joint without impingement. Is is also important to visualize the most anterior medial aspect of the posterior facet to confirm adequate resection.[59] A spacer may be inserted into the former coalition, similar to that for a calcaneonavicular bar. The literature demonstrates excellent success with this. Initially it was thought that if greater than 50% of the size of the posterior facet was involved, then arthrodesis was necessary. Newer studies have shown that resectional arthroplasty of the coalition can be successful in the short to medium term.[60]

In patients noted with a more severe hindfoot valgus and a middle facet coalition comprising more than 50% of the middle facet, an extra-articular subtalar joint arthrodesis may benefit the patient and prevent stunting of the normal hindfoot development. In pediatric patients, fusion of the subtalar joint should be thoroughly discussed, and caution should be taken because of possible growth disturbances of the hindfoot complex.[61] Therefore, the Grice procedure, which was originally described in 1952 as a treatment of children with polio, may be used.[3] The Grice procedure describes an extra-articular subtalar joint arthrodesis that does not affect bone growth in the pediatric patient and has been used to correct spastic valgus deformity in children.[62,63] Although the procedure is not commonly used today, neurologic patients with notable talocalcaneal coalition involving more than 50% of the subtalar joint middle facet and severe spastic hindfoot valgus may benefit.

If there are degenerative changes within the posterior facet, then arthrodesis is warranted. Arthrodesis may also be warranted if the heel valgus is significant. Arthrodesis can be performed from a medial and/or lateral approach. The senior authors'

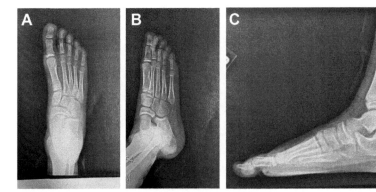

**Fig. 9.** (*A*) Preoperative anteroposterior image of the right foot showing a calcaneonavicular coalition of an 11-year-old male patient. (*B*) Preoperative medial oblique image of the right foot showing a calcaneonavicular coalition of an 11-year-old male patient. Note the narrowing of the calcaneonavicular joint with a fibro-osseous bride limiting motion of the midtarsal joint. (*C*) Preoperative lateral image of the right foot showing a calcaneonavicular coalition of an 11-year-old male patient. Note the "anteater sign" of the anterior process of the calcaneus.

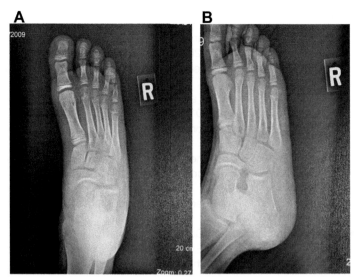

**Fig. 10.** (*A*) Postoperative anteroposterior image of the right foot showing calcaneonavicular coalition resection of an 11-year-old male patient. (*B*) Postoperative medial oblique image of the right foot showing calcaneonavicular coalition resection of an 11-year-old male patient. Note the increase in joint space of the calcaneonavicular joint with no fibro-osseous bridging.

approach is usually a 2-incision approach. Medial incision is used to resect out the middle facet. Lateral sinus tarsi incision is then used to resect the articular cartilage from the posterior facet. Arthrodesis is performed with two 6.5-mm or equivalent screws crossing the subtalar joint.

With resection as well as fusion, additional procedures may be performed as needed. Adjunct procedures may include a medial displacement calcaneal osteotomy, cotton osteotomy, gastrocnemius recession, or an Evans calcaneal osteotomy.

## CLINICS CARE POINTS

- Children and adolescents presenting with multiple ankle sprains should undergo a workup for tarsal coalition.

- Plain radiographs, including calcaneal axial images are paramount. Advanced imaging is ordered to evaluate the extent of the coalition. If differential diagnosis is a fibrous coalition, then MRI is the advanced modality of choice. If an osseous coalition is evaluated, CT evaluation is best.

- Primary surgical intervention of a calcaneonavicular bar is excision as it is an extra-articular coalition. Excision of a middle facet coalition should also include a subtalar joint arthrodesis if subtalar joint degenerative changes are noted.

## DISCLOSURE

G. Golshteyn has nothing to disclose. H.P. Schneider is a consultant for Smith and Nephew.

## REFERENCES

1. Leonard MA. The inheritance of tarsal coalition and its relation to spastic flat foot. J Bone Joint Surg Br 1974;56B:520–6.
2. Stormont DM, Peterson HA. The relative incidence of tarsal coalition. Clin Orthop Relat Res 1983;181:28–36.
3. Khoshbin A, Law PW, Caspi L, et al. Long-term functional outcomes of resected tarsal coalitions. Foot Ankle Int 2013;34(10):1370–5.
4. Harris RI, Beth T. Etiology of peroneal spastic flat foot. J Bone Joint surg 1948; 30B:624–34.
5. Mosca VS, Bevan WP. Talocalcaneal tarsal coalitions and the calcaneal lengthening osteotomy: the role of deformity correction. J Bone Joint Surg 1984;66A: 976–84.
6. Holl M. Beitrage zur chirurgischen osteologie des Fusses. Langenbecks Arch 1880;25:211–23.
7. Bohne W. FACS tarsal coalition. Curr Opin Pediatr 2001;13(1):29–35.
8. Banks AS, Downey MS, Martin DE, et al. McGlamry's comprehensive textbook of foot and ankle surgery, vol. 1. Philadelphia, PA: Lippincott Williams & Wilkins; 2001.
9. Kirmisson E. Double ped bot varus par malformation osseuse primitive associe a des anyloses congenitals des doigs et des orteilze quarte membres d'une meme familee. Rev Orthop 1898;9:392–8.
10. Slomann HC. On coalition calcaneo-navicularis. J Orthop Surg 1921;3:586–602.
11. Cruveilhier A. Anatomie pathologique du corps humain, vol 1. Paris: JB Bailliere; 1829.
12. Badgley CE. Coalition of the calcaneus and navicular. Arch Surg 1927;15:75–88.
13. Lahey MD, Zindrick MR, Harris EJ. A comparative study of the clinical presentation of tarsal coalitions. Clin Podiatric Med Surg 1988;5(2):341–57.
14. Resnik C, Aiken M, Kenzora J. Case report 780. Skeletal Radiol 1993;22(3): 214–7.
15. Zuckerlandl E. Uber einen fall von synostose zwischen talus and calcaneus. Allgemeine Weine Med Zeitung 1877;22:293–4.
16. Korvin H. Coalitio talocanea. Z Orthop Chir 1934;60:105–10.
17. Pfitzner W. Die variationem im aufban des fusskelets. Morphol Arbeit 1896;6: 245–57.
18. Ehrlich MG, Elmer EB. Tarsal coalition. In: Jahss M, editor. Disorders of the foot and ankle. 2nd edition. Philadelphia: W.B. Saunders; 1991. p. 921–38.
19. Solger B. Ueber abnorme verschmelzung knorpeliger skettheile beim fotus. Cent Allgemeine Pathol Patholog Anat 1980;1:124–6.
20. Harris B. Anomalous structure in the developing human foot [Abstract]. Anat Rec 1955;121:399.
21. Harris RI. Rigid valgus foot due to talocalcaneal bridge. J Bone Joint Surg. 1955; 37A:169–83.
22. Boyd H. Congenital talonavicular synostosis. J Bone Joint Surg 1944;26:682.
23. Wray J, Herndon C. Hereditary transmission of congenital coalition of the calcaneus to the navicular. J Bone Joint Surg 1963;45-A:293.
24. Menz HB. Two feet, or one person? Problems associated with statistical analysis of paired data in foot and ankle medicine. Foot 2004;14:2–5.
25. Sullivan RJ. Adolescent foot and ankle conditions. Orthopedic knowledge update: foot and ankle. Am Acad Orthop Surg 2008;4:48–50.

26. Snyder RB, Lipscomb AB, Johnston RK. The relationship of tarsal coalitions to ankle sprains in athletes. Am J Sports Med 1981;9(5):313–7.
27. Jack EA. Bone anomalies of the tarsus in relation to "peroneal spastic flat foot. J Bone Joint Surg Br 1954;36-B(4):530–42.
28. Mosca VS. Subtalar coalition in pediatrics. Foot Ankle Clin 2015;20:265–81.
29. Lapidus PW. Spastic flat foot. J Bone Joint Surg Am 1946;28:126–36.
30. Outland T, Murphy ID. The pathomechanics of peroneal spastic flat foot. Clin Orthop 1960;16:64–73.
31. Schmidt F. Uber eine symmetrische synostosis calcaneo navicularis bei gleichzeitigem klumphohlfuss. Arch F Orthop U Unfall-Chir 1931;30:289.
32. Cass AD, Camasta CA. A review of tarsal coalition and pes planovalgus: clinical examination, diagnostic imaging, and surgical planning. J Foot Ankle Surg 2010; 49:274–93.
33. Lowy LJ. Pediatric peroneal spastic flatfoot in the absence of coalition: a suggested protocol. J Am Podiatr Med Assoc 1998;88(4):181–91.
34. Lyon R, Liu X, Cho S. Effect of tarsal coalition resection on dynamic plantar pressures and electromyography of lower extremity muscles. J Foot Ankle Surg 2005; 44(4):252–8.
35. Yu GV. Asymptomatic tarsal coalitions. In: Ruch JA, Vickers NS, Camasta CA, editors. Reconstructive surgery of the foot and leg, update 1993. Tucker, GA: The Podiatry Institute; 1993. p. 246–55.
36. Downey MS, Rich JA. Juvenile peroneal spastic flatfoot-tarsal coalitions. In: McGlamry ED, editor. Doctors hospital podiatric education and research fourteenth annual surgical sminar syllabus. Atlanta: Doctors Hospital Podiatry Institute; 1985. p. 56.
37. Conway JJ, Cowell HR. Tarsal coalition: clinical significance and roentgenographic demonstration. Radiology 1969;92(4):799–811.
38. Downey MS. Tarsal coalition: current clinical aspects with introduction of a surgical classification. In: McGlamry ED, editor. Reconstructive surgery of the foot and leg: update '89. Tucker, GA: Podiatry Institute; 1989. p. 60–700.
39. Newman JS, Newberg AH. Congenital tarsal coalition: multimodality evaluation with emphasis on CT and MR imaging. Radiographics 2000;20:321–32.
40. Cowell HR. Talocacaneal coalition and new causes of peroneal spastic flatfoot. Clin Orthop 1972;85:16–22.
41. Cowell HR. Talocalcaneal coalition and new causes of peroneal spastic flatfoot. Clin Orthop Relat Res 1972;85:16–22.
42. Blakemore LC, Cooperman DR, Thompson GH. The rigid flatfoot: tarsal coalitions. Clin Pod Med Surg 2000;17(3):531–55.
43. Katayama T, Tanaka Y, Kadono K, et al. Talocalcaneal coalition: a case showing the ossification process. Foot Ankle Int 2005;26(6):490–3.
44. Kumai T, Takahura Y, Akiyama K, et al. Histopathological study of nonosseous tarsal coalition. Foot Ankle Int 1998;19(8):525–31.
45. Haddad SL, Deland JT. Pes planus. Mann's Surgery of the Foot and Ankle. vol. 1. 9th edition. Philadelphia: Saunders; 2014. Chapter: 25. p. 1349–51.
46. Brown RR, Rosenberg ZS, Thornhill BA. The C sign: more specific for flatfoot deformity than subtalar coalition. Skeletal Radiol 2001;30(2):84–7.
47. Newman JS, Newberg AH. Congenital tarsal coalition: multimodality evaluation with emphasis on CT and MR Imaging. Radiographics 2000;2013:321–32.
48. Varich L, Bancroft L. Radiologic case study. Talocalcaneal coalition. Orthopedics 2010;2013:374–452.

49. Oestreich AE, Mize WA, Crawford AH, et al. The "anteater nose": a direct sign of calcaneonavicular coalition on the lateral radiograph. J Pediatr Orthop 1987;7(6): 709–11.
50. Carson CW, Ginsburg WW, Cohen MD, et al. Tarsal coalition: an unusual cause of foot pain—clinical spectrum and treatment in 129 patients. Semin Arthritis Rheum 1991;20(6):367–77.
51. Crim JE, Kjeldsberg KM. Radiographc diagnosis of tarsal coalitions. AJR Am J Roentgenol 2004;182:323–8.
52. Emery KH, Bisset GS 3rd, Johnson ND, et al. Tarsal coalition: a blinded comparison of MRI and CT. Pediatr Radiol 1998;28:612–6.
53. Rocchi V, Huang MT, Bomar JD, et al. The "double medial malleolus": a new physical finding in talocalcaneal coalition. J Pediatr Orthop 2018;38(4):239–43.
54. Perlman MD, Wertheimer SJ. Tarsal coalitions. J Foot Surg 1986;25:58.
55. Downey MS. Tarsal coalitions, A surgical classification. J Am Podiatr Med Assoc 1991;81(4):187–97.
56. Tachdjian MO. The childs foot. Philadelphia: WB Saunders; 1985. p. 261–94.
57. Shirley E, Gheorghe R, Neal K. Results of nonoperative treatment for symptomatic tarsal coalitions. Cureus 2018;10(7):e2944.
58. Badgley CE. Coalition of the calcaneus and the navicular. Arch Surg 1927;15:75.
59. Gantsoudes GD, Roocroft JH, Mubarak SJ. Treatment of talocalcaneal coalitions. J Pediatr Orthop 2012;32(3):301–7.
60. Luhmann SJ, Schoenecker PL. Symptomatic talocalcaneal coalition resection: indications and results. J Pediatr Orthop 1998;18:748–54.
61. Zhou B, Tang K, Hardy M. Talocalcaneal coalition combined with flatfoot in children: diagnosis and treatment: a review. J Orthop Surg Res 2014;9:129.
62. Grice DS. Ax extra-articular arthrodesis of the subastragalar. Joint 1952;34: 927–56.
63. Høiness PR, Kirkhus E. Grice arthrodesis in the treatment of valgus feet in children with myelomeningocele: a 12.8-year follow-up study. J Child Orthop 2009; 3:283–90.

# Gradual Correction of Pediatric Equinus Deformity

Lucian M. Feraru, DPM*, Mark E. Solomon, DPM

## KEYWORDS

- Neurologic Equinus • Marfan's syndrome • Charcot–Marie–Tooth
- Pediatric equinus • Gradual correction • External fixation

## KEY POINTS

- Pediatric equinus is associated with pathology of bone, soft tissue or a combined deformity.
- Rigid plantarflexed cases can be debilitating to the point of inability to ambulate.
- It is important to obtain a thorough history from the parents and to perform a comprehensive physical examination that includes the foot and ankle as well as a superstructural evaluation.
- Treatments always begin with conservative management such as stretching and progress to possible surgery for lengthening of the Achilles tendon or gastrocnemius release.
- Gradual correction via external fixation is a viable option for rigid, recalcitrant cases where previous surgery has failed.

## INTRODUCTION

Pediatric equinus is broadly defined as generalized limited dorsiflexion at the ankle joint. It may result from either congenital or acquired causes and exhibit varying characteristics such as flexible, rigid, or spastic types. It has been extensively studied in the literature and is known to be associated with the pathological condition of the bone, soft tissue, or combined deformity. In children, rigid plantarflexed cases can be debilitating and prevent them from ambulating without pain, if at all. As this volume in Clinics has articles on comprehensive pediatric examination and neuromuscular disorders, this article will focus on (non-neurologic equinus)

- Congenital causes
  - Intrauterine stroke, phocomelia, hemimelia

---

The Pediatric Orthopedic Fellowship, 218 Ridgedale Avenue #101, Cedar Knolls, NJ 07927, USA
* Corresponding author.
*E-mail address:* lucian.m.feraru@gmail.com

Clin Podiatr Med Surg 39 (2022) 143–156
https://doi.org/10.1016/j.cpm.2021.09.006
0891-8422/22/© 2021 Elsevier Inc. All rights reserved.

- Acquired causes
  - Trauma, neoplasm, infection, burn, compartment syndrome, prolonged immobilization after NV accident)
- Idiopathic
  - Autism, sensory integration issues

### History

History is paramount to identifying the cause and formulating a treatment of equinus. Questions that should be asked include the time of onset, percentage of time spent on toes, ability of the patient to get their heels on the ground at all during gait or stance, any previous workup or interventions (conservative or surgical) as well as the presence of toe walking in the family history.[1]
Questions to ask parents.

- Is there family history of developmental dysplasia of hip, neuromuscular disease (muscular dystrophy), any hereditary conditions such as Charcot–Marie–Tooth, any spastic paralyses, scoliosis, connective tissue disease such as Marfan's syndrome, neurofibromatosis
- Neonatal history
- Developmental history/milestones
- Patient's normal activity level
- Are there any neurologic symptoms such as radiating pain, loss of bowel or bladder control?
- Onset time of toe walking, percentage of time spent on toes, ability to get heels on ground during gait/stance
- Any previous workup or interventions and relevant findings?

Toe walking is often seen as a complaint on presentation identified by the family. Milder, nonneurologic forms resolve around the age of 3. Heel contact increases once walking ability improves. Typically, the parental concern is noted when toe walking continues as most of the peers are achieving heel strike. Idiopathic toe walking is a diagnosis of exclusion, after all, other causes of a similar gait pattern have been ruled out. If no musculoskeletal or neurologic etiology is identified, the condition may improve spontaneously.[2]
Orthopedic pathologies such as clubfoot, developmental hip dysplasia, as well as knee and hip flexion contractures can play a role in the equinus development. To properly assess a toe walking child, physical examination should be comprehensive, with a high level of attention to the musculoskeletal system, reaching milestones, and gait. The diagnostic workup should include a referral to a neurodevelopmental pediatrician for a more in-depth evaluation.[1]

### Clinical examination

#### Static: standing: front, back, and both sides

General
- Limb length discrepancy – Use wood blocks ranging from 0.5 cm to 6 cm until pelvis is level
Head/neck
- Head tilt and rotation
- Facies – evaluate cleft palate, synostosis, syndromic
Shoulders
- Uneven shoulder or scapula levels

Cervical/thoracic spine
- Scoliosis or kyphosis

Pelvis
- ASIS symmetry and level

Knee joint
- Knee deformity in all 3 planes.
- Patella position.

Ankle joint
- Ankle equinus
- Calcaneus deformity from the side

Hindfoot
- Varus or valgus from the back

Mid/forefoot
- Forefoot or toe deformity.
- In-toe/out-toe

### Static: sitting: front, back, and both sides

General
Head/neck
- Head tilt and rotation
- Manipulate - active and passive movements
- Facies - cleft palate, synostosis/syndromic

Lumbar spine
- Lumbar lordosis suggestive of flexion deformity of the hip when the patient is supine on a hard surface

Pelvis
- ASIS level and symmetry

Hip joint
- Manipulate – active and passive ROM

Knee joint
- Knee deformity in all 3 planes.
- Patella position.
- Manipulate - active and passive movements ROM

Ankle joint
- Ankle equinus
- Calcaneus deformity from the side

Hindfoot
- Varus or valgus from the back

Mid/forefoot
- Forefoot or toe deformity.
- In-toe/out-toe

### Static: prone: front, back, and both sides

Head/neck
- Head and tilt rotation
- Manipulate – active and passive movements
- Facies - cleft palate, synostosis/syndromic

Lumbar spine
- Lumbar lordosis suggestive of flexion deformity of the hip when the patient is supine on a hard surface

Pelvis
- ASIS level and symmetry

Hip joint
- Manipulate – active and passive ROM

Thigh/femur
- Evaluate femoral anteversion: *Craig's test*
  - Joint position – knee flexed to 90°.
  - Procedure- One hand of the examiner is placed flat on the greater trochanter. Hold the leg and gently rotate the hip in both directions till the greater trochanter is maximally prominent. The amount of internal rotation needed to make the greater trochanter maximally prominent is the degree of anteversion.
  - In addition, the range of rotational movement of the hip is also recorded. The patient is made prone and the pelvis is made level. Then rotate the hip internally and externally to the maximum point to which it is maintained by gravity alone. In patients with excessive femoral anteversion, the range of internal rotation is increased, and external rotation is diminished. In femoral retroversion, the external rotation is increased and internal rotation diminished.

Knee joint
- Knee deformity in all 3 planes.
- Patella position.
- Manipulate - active and passive movements ROM

Leg/tibia
- Tibial torsion: First evaluate foot for metatarsus adductus using *Bleck's line.*
- If foot normal:
  - Thigh foot angle is assessed by the following method.
  - Joint position – knee flexed to 90°, ankle in the neutral position.
  - Procedure – measure the angle between the thigh axis and the foot axis. Angle is negative if internally rotated and positive if externally rotated. Normally the angle is 10° in adults. In the newborn, there is 5° internal tibial torsion normally.
- If foot abnormal and metatarsus adductus present:
  - Pt is prone with knee flexed to 90.
  - The pointer and index fingers are placed on the distal aspect of the malleoli. A line should be drawn or perceived between these 2 points. This is compared with the longitudinal axis of the thigh.

Ankle joint
- Ankle equinus
- Calcaneus deformity from the side

Hindfoot
- Varus or valgus from the back

Mid/forefoot
- Forefoot or toe deformity.
- In-toe/out-toe.

### Static: supine: front, back, and both sides

Head/neck
- Head and tilt rotation
- Manipulate – active and passive movements
- Facies - cleft palate, synostosis/syndromic

Lumbar spine
- Lumbar lordosis suggestive of flexion deformity of the hip when the patient is supine on a hard surface.

- If present, do the Thomas test to assess the severity of flexion deformity.
  - Thomas test:
  - Examiner position – Stand on the right side of the patient with one hand under the lumbar spine of the patient. With the other hand hold the unaffected side.
  - Procedure- Flex the unaffected knee fully, then flex the unaffected hip till the excessive lumbar lordosis disappears. Measure the angle between the thigh of the affected side and the table to assess the angle of fixed flexion deformity of the hip.

Pelvis
- ASIS level and symmetry

Hip joint
- Manipulate – active and passive ROM

Knee joint
- Knee deformity in all 3 planes.
- Patella position.

Ankle joint
- Ankle equinus
- Calcaneus deformity from the side

Hindfoot
- Varus or valgus from the back

Mid/forefoot
- Forefoot or toe deformity.
- In-toe/out-toe

## GAIT/DYNAMIC: FRONT, BACK, AND BOTH SIDES

General
- Limb length discrepancy

Head/neck
- Head and tilt rotation

Shoulders
- Uneven shoulder or scapula levels

Pelvis
- ASIS level and symmetry

Knee joint
- Knee deformity in all 3 planes.
- Patella position.

Ankle joint
- Ankle equinus
- Calcaneus deformity from the side

Hindfoot
- Varus or valgus from the back
- Toe-walking – does it change on different floor textures or temperatures?

Mid/forefoot
- Forefoot or toe deformity.
- In-toe/out-toe: Foot progression angle is the angular difference between the direction of walking and the long axis of the foot. If the foot is externally rotated, then the angle is positive and if internally rotated then the angle is negative. Normal value for children and adolescents is 10°.

It is important to avoid getting tunnel vision when evaluating equinus and consider any superstructural issue above the ankle. Mechanical alignment of the lower extremity is based on the additive effects of the bony alignment between the femur, tibia, and foot as well as the influence by the hip, knee, and ankle joints. A comprehensive examination should include static and dynamic phases of inspection, palpation, manipulation of joints/range of motion, and special testing. The patient should be observed standing, sitting, walking, and in the prone and supine positions. The examiner should evaluate from the front, back, and both sides. The goal is to identify any primary or secondary structural points of asymmetry, local or regional components, and compensatory changes.

Initial observation should begin when the child is walking to the examination room, unaware that they are being observed. If possible, the patient should be wearing shorts and a shirt so the examiner is unencumbered by bulky clothing, yet modesty should be observed. The author begins the examination in whichever position will make the patient the most comfortable and cooperative. Depending on the age, it is sometimes best to perform an examination with child alongside or sitting in the parent's lap. The dynamic examination can be performed afterward with the parent waiting at the end of a hallway. Acquiring good reliable data are often directly proportional to the patience and flexibility of the examiner.

## INSPECTION

Key findings should include: LLD. Look for any asymmetry in size, shape, and function. Assess for muscle wasting.

## PALPATION

Palpate the bone, soft tissues, and joint. Look for change in temperature; limb with post-polio residual contracture is cold. Look for any tenderness and note the site of tenderness. When palpating bony and soft tissues; look for any asymmetry, thickening, swelling, or defect.

## MANIPULATION/JOINT RANGE OF MOTION

Assess the active and passive movements of spine, hip, knee, foot, and ankle.

Look for the restriction of range of movement, pain during joint movement, ligamentous laxity, joint instability, and any abnormal sounds during joint movement.

While moving the joint passively, watch out for muscle spasm.

Movement should be assessed in all 3 planes depending on the normal movement for that particular joint.

## SPECIAL TESTING

LLD: Limb length discrepancy may be true or functional. True LLD is due to real shortening or lengthening. Functional LLD is due to abnormal joint positioning such as the adduction contracture of the hip. Limb length discrepancy (LLD) may be true or functional. True LLD is due to the shortening or lengthening of bone or joint dislocation. Functional LLD is due to the abnormal joint positioning such as pelvic obliquity due to the adduction contracture or flexion deformity of knee.

When the patient is standing; assess whether the shoulder, iliac crest, and the popliteal and gluteal creases are at the same level. Look for compensatory scoliosis, which will disappear if the patient is made to sit. LLD may be masked by flexion of the opposite knee and plantar flexion of ankle.

With measuring tape; measure both the true length and apparent length. Apparent length is measured from the xiphisternum or umbilicus to the inferior tip of the medial malleolus when the limbs are kept parallel. To measure the true length, both the limbs should be kept in an identical position. Hence if there is a fixed adduction deformity of hip; first make the pelvis level by adducting the affected hip till both the anterior superior iliac spines (ASIS) are at the same level. Measure the true length of the affected limb from the inferior edge of ASIS to the inferior edge of the medial malleolus. Now keep the opposite hip also in an identical degree of adduction and then measure the other side as well.

## TORSIONAL/ROTATIONAL ABNORMALITIES

Pediatric equinus may present with either a primary or secondary component hidden within a torsional or rotational abnormality. This may occur within the spine, pelvis, femur, tibia, foot, or combination thereof. The gait will either present as in-toeing, out-toeing, or a windswept deformity in which one limb will point in and the contralateral limb will point outwards. These are highly complex deformities that most likely present with an LLD as well.

## ANGULAR DEFORMITY

Ask the patient to stand with his feet and knee touching each other while the patella is facing forwards. When inspected from the front, there will be a gap between the knees in patients with genu varum. In patients with genu valgum, the ankles will be kept apart. Inspect from the side, specifically looking for equinus or calcaneus deformity of ankle, flexion deformity, or hyperextension deformity of knee.

In addition, measure the intercondylar distance between medial femoral condyles in the standing position for genu varum. In cases of genu valgum measure the intermalleolar distance in the standing position.

Intercondylar distance is measured to assess the severity of genu varum deformity. Ask the patient to stand with his medial malleoli touching each other and then measure the distance between the medial femoral condyles. Intermalleolar distance is measured in patients with genu valgum deformity. Ask the patient to stand with his medial femoral condyles touching each other and the foot should be in neutral rotation, measure the distance between the medial malleoli. Both these measurements have the disadvantage of being influenced by the size of the patient. In this situation, measurement of the tibiofemoral angle using a goniometer is essential. This is measured in the standing position. Lateral thigh leg angle is measured by keeping the arms of the goniometer on the lateral surface of thigh and leg and the hinge of the goniometer at the level of knee. Another method is by keeping the arms of goniometer on the anterior surface of the thigh and leg and the hinge of the goniometer over the center of patella.

In patients with genu valgum one should do the Ober's test to rule out ITB contracture and assess the patient for patellofemoral instability. Measure the standing height, sitting height, and arm span of the patient.

Thomas' test is used to evaluate hip flexion. Joint contractures for the hip are described as $\geq 20°$ of contracture, for the knee it is $\geq 20°$ of contracture, and for the ankle it is $\geq 15°$ of fixed ankle equinus. Contractures of the hip and knee may go unrecognized which can lead to recurrence, as well as knee or hip dislocations. It is recommended to treat hip and knee pathological conditions before intervention at the level of the ankle.[3]

The Silfverskiöld test is used to examine ankle joint dorsiflexion with knee extended and flexed. If the patient has less than 5° of ankle joint dorsiflexion with the knee extended, but greater than 10° of ankle joint dorsiflexion with the knee flexed, then the patient has gastrocnemius equinus. If the patient has less than 10° of ankle dorsiflexion with knee flexed, then they have gastrocnemius-soleus equinus. There is controversy regarding the necessary amount of ankle dorsiflexion during the stance phase of gait; however, 3 to 15° of ankle motion past perpendicular is generally accepted with the knee extended.[4]

## RADIOGRAPHIC DETERMINATION OF EQUINUS DEFORMITY

Weight-bearing radiographs can be performed by a number of different methods, including a limb length scan-o-gram or an EOS scan. The previously measured height of wooden blocks should be used to level the limbs and reduce measurement errors due to pelvic obliquity or torsional compensation. The patellae should be forward facing to reveal any hidden issues. The frontal and sagittal planes should be evaluated for total limb length and the heights of the pelvic, femoral, tibial, and foot segments. The joints should also be evaluated for soft tissue laxity or compensation.

### Treatment Options

Both conservative and surgical treatments have been described for pediatric equinus. If the condition is flexible, stretching may be enough. In recalcitrant cases, soft tissue procedures such as a tendo-Achilles lengthening (TAL), gastrocnemius recession, or even a posterior capsular release have been reported with varying outcomes. Even with cases that present with rigid equinus, it is the Author's preference to always exhaust conservative options before proceeding to surgery.

For patients with idiopathic toe walking, the Cincinnati care guidelines were developed to guide treatment based on patient age and severity of toe walking. Nonsurgical treatments are first used, consisting of physical therapy with stretching, strengthening, gait training, and home exercise. Serial casting, ankle-foot orthoses as well as nighttime splints may be attempted. Surgical treatments consist of TAL or gastrocnemius recession.[1]

In patients younger than age 11, serial casting is recommended for patients with 0° of ankle dorsiflexion. Ideally, this is performed in the office by an experienced Ponseti practitioner. Hopefully, this results in about 5° of dorsiflexion which is discontinued once the patient reaches 5° to 10° of passive dorsiflexion. If the patient already has 5° of dorsiflexion, they can attempt physical therapy and gait training as well as nighttime stretching. This can be set up as a home program by skilled physical therapy or health care professional. If the patient presents with 5° to 10° of ankle dorsiflexion, treatment is similar, with frequency and duration individualized to each patient. Treatment should be continued until the patient improves balance, ankle dorsiflexion, heel gait pattern with or without AFO.[1]

Botulinum injection has been studied as a treatment of spastic equinus, showing significant improvements in gait after multiple injections. Metxiotis and colleagues studied 47 children with cerebral palsy which received between 2 and 4 botulinum injections and no casting. The authors recommend injections every 4 to 6 months to minimize antibody formation and financial burden of therapy, allowing for a delay in the need for orthopedic surgery.[5] Glanzman and colleagues suggest using botulinum before serial casting as a means to reduce treatment time and number of casts, and have shown improved passive dorsiflexion in patients receiving casting and injections versus injections alone.[6]

Many open soft tissue surgical procedures have been described. The Bauman procedure is performed through a medial incision and resects the aponeurosis overlying the anterior aspect of the gastrocnemius. The greatest structures at risk for this procedure are the saphenous nerve and the greater saphenous vein. Strayer described the open release more distally at the musculotendinous junction of the gastrocnemius. The sural nerve is most at risk during this procedure. The Strayer can also be performed as an endoscopic procedure, with increased risk of sural neuropraxia. The Vulpius procedure has been described and is often used for children with spastic diplegia. This procedure is performed distal to the musculotendinous junction and lengthens both the gastrocnemius and the soleus muscles.[2]

## GRADUAL CORRECTION

Gradual correction is indicated in situations whereby previous surgery has failed. It allows deformity correction through minimal incisions which reduce the risk of scarring or further damage to soft tissues. It allows fine tuning of the deformity correction, as well as joint range of motion and early ambulation while the frame protects and stress shields the surgical sites. Using gradual correction reduces the risk of affecting the Blix contractile curve. This is because muscle fibers have been shown to lengthen via sarcomere addition, which allows sarcomeres to remain at the optimal length to provide the strongest contraction, resulting in the maintenance of muscle strength. Acute muscle lengthening, however, may result in permanent muscle weakness. Another advantage of external fixation is the reduced need to perform talectomy or triple arthrodesis which is disabling to the pediatric population. Gradual correction may obviate the need for soft tissue expanders, extensive soft tissue release, shortening osteotomies as well as free-tissue transfer flaps. It also reduces morbidity associated with large deformity correction when dealing with burns, scars, and skin with poor protoplasm. Acute correction has a higher risk of neurovascular compromise, which can be avoided with controlled gradual correction. Lamm and colleagues often perform prophylactic tarsal tunnel release before or during correction of equinus greater than 10 to 20°, especially if there is a concomitant varus deformity. Typically, children under the age of 8 still possess biological plasticity which allows their deformity to be corrected using only soft tissue and joint distraction. This can be compared with serial casting treatment in infants. Stretching stiff tissues as opposed to surgically releasing them reduces the risk of scarring and intraarticular fibrosis. Children above the age of 8 will likely need distraction osteogenesis.

Gradual correction of pediatric equinus deformity can be accomplished only after extensive deformity analysis and planning have been achieved. The surgery consists of two phases, the initial stage corrects the underlying deformity and the latter stage involves both restoration and preservation of the ankle joint range of motion. Length of correction depends on the degree of initial equinus plus a residual program to overcorrect to 10 to 15 dorsiflexion. The rate of correction is at a maximum angular correction of 2° per day.

Overcorrected deformity should be maintained for approximately 4 to 6 weeks. Depending on the patient circumstances and surgeon's preference to perform adjunctive soft tissue correction, the overall duration may be reduced. After removing the external fixator, apply a long leg cast to maintain overcorrected position. A custom AFO should be worn for the first 6 months. Tendon transfers/balancing may be considered if dynamic recurrence or motor imbalance is noted. If recurrence is rigid, osteotomies may be necessary and/or arthrodesis.

It is important to differentiate soft tissue contractures from skeletal abnormalities. Ankle equinus can be mimicked by distal tibial procurvatum, forefoot equinus as well as a flat-top talus. These osseous deformities can coexist with soft tissue contractures.

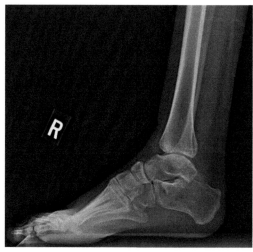

**Fig. 1.** Preoperative radiographs showing an Anterior Distal Tibial Angle (ADTA) of 91° and a Tibial Sole Angle of 101°. A bone block is noted secondary to procurvatum.

Fixators used in the correction of equinus can have a uniaxial hinge (constrained) or may have no hinge (unconstrained). The Taylor-Spatial Frame construct has a virtual hinge and is typically used for correction of multiaxial, multijoint deformities such as clubfoot. Constrained fixators will have a single hinge centered through the axis of the ankle joint. This construct allows a range of motion during correction of the contracture. It is important to apply fixation to the calcaneus and talus to avoid over the distraction of the subtalar joint. Physiolysis is a spontaneous fracture of the distal tibial physis which can occur during distraction. Placing a wire transversely through the distal tibial epiphysis and connected to the tibial block can help stabilize the growth plate.

Toe flexion contractures may occur during the correction, which is a result of extrinsic toe flexor tightening. Toes can be kept stretched using toe slings made of leather in combination with elastic bands attached to the frame. Toe splints can be molded and held to the fixator using Velcro straps. Physical therapy performed regularly will help prevent stiffness and contractures. If contractures are preexisting, a percutaneous flexor release can be performed at the plantar digital crease. In older children, wires can be advanced through the toes individually which can gradually pull them upward or maintain them in a corrected position.

Disadvantages of external fixation include the need for high surgical expertise, complications such as pin site infections are common, there is a risk for disuse osteopenia even when using walking rings.[4,7,8]

Pediatric equinus is a common disorder with extensive literature on identification and treatment of the condition. Serial casting is always indicated as a first-line conservative treatment unless the deformity is completely rigid. For the more complex cases, external fixation has been reported as a safe, effective technique for gradual correction.

## CASE REPORT

A 15 year old female presented to the office for recurrence of Talipes Equinovarus of the right lower extremity. She has been complaining of pain and disability as a result of

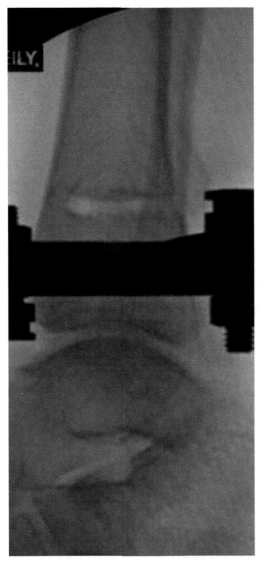

**Fig. 2.** Opening tibial osteotomy with anterior hinge performed using a drill and continuous irrigation to minimize bony necrosis.

the fixed equinus. She underwent Ponseti casting in the Dominican Republic at 13 days old and a TAL was performed at 8 years of age with success to her left side. A Tendo Achilles lengthening was attempted in 2019 for the right side, with no resolution. Upon evaluation of her right lower extremity, she had no hip or knee contractures. Heel bisection is 4th toe however flexible to neutral. She is in a rigid equinus position. Approximately 10 mm of limb length discrepancy was noted with the right side being shorter. She was exhibiting a circumduction gait with the right ankle in equinus. **Fig. 1** shows preoperative lateral radiograph.

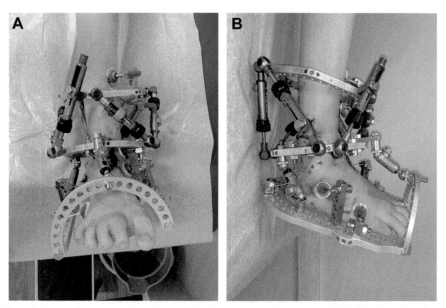

**Fig. 3.** Immediate postoperative clinical pictures showing tibial block with hex configuration.

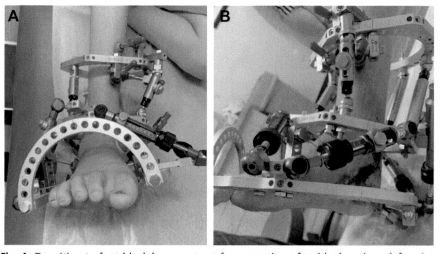

**Fig. 4.** Transition to foot block hex construct for correction of residual equinus deformity.

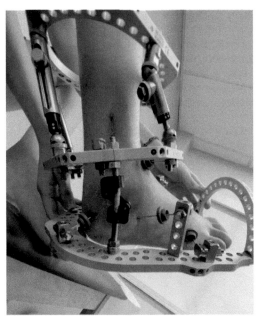

**Fig. 5.** Lateral view with hinges along Inman's axis allowing range of motion of the ankle joint.

The procedure consisted of a tarsal tunnel release with an abductor fascial release, a distal tibia-fibular metaphyseal osteotomy, an application of a multiplanar external fixator with stereotactic computer assisted adjustments, and finally resection of the talar neck osteophyte. (**Fig. 2**) Gradual correction was performed at a rate of maximum 2 degrees per day, with four adjustments per day. (**Fig. 3**) After the correction program was completed, the proximal block was converted to static struts and the hex struts were applied to the foot block to attain soft tissue correction of the residual equinus. (**Fig. 4**) After this was achieved, the foot block was converted to a hinge mechanism to allow ankle range of motion and ambulation through the frame. (**Fig. 5**) This will maintain protection of the osteotomy site until full consolidation is noted. At that time, the frame is removed and an aggressive physical therapy regimen is employed to help maintain range of motion and allow full weight bearing and a return to function.

## REFERENCES

1. Bennett JF, Omura J. Toe walking: review of the differential diagnosis and treatment options to ensure optimal gross motor development. PA Clin 2020;5(4): 477–85.

2. Solan MC, Kohls-Gatzoulis J, Stephens MM. Idiopathic toe walking and contractures of the triceps surae. Foot Ankle Clin 2010;15(2):297–307.

3. Bartlett MD, Wolf LS, Shurtleff DB, et al. Hip flexion contractures: a comparison of measurement methods. Arch Phys Med Rehabil 1985;66(9):620–5. PMID: 4038029.

4. Lamm BM, Standard SC, Galley IJ, et al. External fixation for the foot and ankle in children. Clin Podiatr Med Surg 2006;23(1):137–66.

5. Metaxiotis D, Siebel A, Doederlein L. Repeated botulinum toxin A injections in the treatment of spastic equinus foot. Clin Orthop Relat Res 2002;394:177–85.
6. Glanzman AM, Kim H, Swaminathan K, et al. Efficacy of botulinum toxin A, serial casting, and combined treatment for spastic equinus: a retrospective analysis. Dev Med Child Neurol 2004;46(12):807–11.
7. Gourdine-Shaw MC, Lamm BM, Herzenberg JE, et al. Equinus deformity in the pediatric patient: causes, evaluation, and management. Clin Podiatr Med Surg 2010; 27(1):25–42.
8. Lindsey CA, Makarov MR, Shoemaker S, et al. The effect of the amount of limb lengthening on skeletal muscle. Clin Orthop Relat Res 2002;402:278–87.

# *Moving?*

## *Make sure your subscription moves with you!*

To notify us of your new address, find your **Clinics Account Number** (located on your mailing label above your name), and contact customer service at:

**Email: journalscustomerservice-usa@elsevier.com**

**800-654-2452** (subscribers in the U.S. & Canada)
**314-447-8871** (subscribers outside of the U.S. & Canada)

**Fax number: 314-447-8029**

**Elsevier Health Sciences Division**
**Subscription Customer Service**
**3251 Riverport Lane**
**Maryland Heights, MO 63043**

ELSEVIER